In A
SPLIT SECOND
Living in the World With Cerebral Palsy

KYLE N. SCOTT

◆ FriesenPress

One Printers Way
Altona, MB R0G0B0,
Canada

www.friesenpress.com

Copyright © 2021 by Kyle N. Scott
First Edition — 2021

All rights reserved.

No part of this publication may be reproduced in any form, or by any means, electronic or mechanical, including photocopying, recording, or any information browsing, storage, or retrieval system, without permission in writing from FriesenPress.

ISBN
978-1-5255-9788-6 (Hardcover)
978-1-5255-9787-9 (Paperback)
978-1-5255-9789-3 (eBook)

1. Biography & Autobiography, Personal Memoirs

Distributed to the trade by The Ingram Book Company

Kyle. N. Scott

Endorsements

A MUST-READ! I couldn't put it down! This memoir is not just for those of us who are physically disabled or who have a family member with this disability; it is for everyone! Through this sensitive and insightful book written in his humorous, yet serious style, Kyle invites us to walk in his shoes (so to speak) and experience his unique life's journey with his family and friends.

Even though my life's work was devoted to the educational journey of individuals with disabilities assisting them to navigate the system and become successful, Kyle's personal journey writings gave me a deeper insight into the daily mixture of emotions, feelings, obstacles, and yes... dare I say chaos often experienced by the individual and their families.

His candour is admirable! His humour is infectious! An enjoyable and informative read!

I couldn't put the book down! This book needs to be read to discover one man's secret to living life to its fullest potential!

Joanne Gera
Retired Department Head of Special Education
Presently Board Chair for Conway Homes: independent living for individuals with physical disabilities
Hamilton, Ontario, Canada

Scott's Split Second provides a window into the psyche of an adult living with CP. Mr. Scott regales the reader with stories of his childhood, school experiences, participation in team sports and experiments in finding love. He shows us the many daily challenges he faces to put his mark on society.

This memoir is a must-read for anyone who wants to understand the thoughts, dreams and perspective of someone living with CP, all while maintaining a sunny, "can-do" attitude against all odds.

Lian Cavarzan, B.A.(Hons), B.Ed., M.A.(T), O.C.T.
Elementary Principal
Hamilton, Ontario, Canada

Kyle Scott willingly puts his vulnerability on display while providing a compelling voice for the cerebral palsy community.

Whether you are living with a disability, a caregiver, friend, family member, educator, inspiration seeker or just want to learn more, Kyle provides insight and many lessons through this candid sharing of his many challenges and successes from birth, childhood, adolescence and into adulthood.

Kyle's memory and attention to detail in his storytelling is remarkable. The love for those who have impacted his journey is undeniable and shines throughout this heartfelt memoir.

In a time when we have been forced to pause, this book is a strong reminder to take stock and appreciate what is most important in life, the unconditional support of family and friends in your village.

Dennis Hamel, B.A., B. Ed.
Elementary Teacher
Burlington, Ontario, Canada

Table of Contents

Endorsements, v

Acknowledgements, ix

Introduction, xiii

Chapter 1: In a Split Second, 1

Chapter 2: Starting School, 13

Chapter 3: High School Life, 25

Chapter 4: College Years, 41

Chapter 5: My Sporting Career, 51

Chapter 6: Living with CP — Emotionally, 73

Chapter 7: Living with CP — Physically, 83

Chapter 8: Dating and Intimacy, 93

Chapter 9: My Faith and Spirituality, 113

Chapter 10: Memories and Celebrations That Will Last a Lifetime, 127

Chapter 11: Trips and Adventures, 159

Chapter 12: Amusing Anecdotes, 189

Chapter 13: With Us in Spirit: Tributes to Family and Friends Who Have Passed, 205

Chapter 14: Poetic Musings, 225

Epilogue, 235

Author's Note, 239

Acknowledgements

To Mom and Dad:

I would like to express my deep gratitude to you for helping me to become the man that I am. From the bottom of my heart, thank you for everything you have done, and continue to do, for Stirling and me. Your unwavering love, care, support, belief, and faith are far beyond anything I could ever desire. I have been blessed with parents who are perfect role models. I love you more than words can ever express.

Thank you for giving me the strength to reach for the stars and chase my dreams. I couldn't have done it without both of you.

I look forward to creating many more cherished moments together in the years to come.

To Stirling:

I couldn't have asked for a more high-spirited and spitfire brother to be a part of my life. I remember the day you were born and when we brought you home; I was extremely thrilled. Well, at least until you started giving me that stern look you give — *a Scott family trait*. Even though there is a six-year gap between us, we still always played with each other in the household. I will always remember the day when you told Dad exactly who you were after being sent to your room. He scolded you for misbehaving, and you turned around and said, "I am your son. I am Kyle's brother. I pay the consequences around here. You go to your room!" You were only three years old at the time and you decided to misuse the word "consequences," probably because it was the biggest word you knew, but everyone couldn't help but laugh at how smart yet stubborn you were at such a young age.

We drifted apart during the pre-teen/teenage years because of our difference in life stages. As an older brother, I wanted to guide you and give you the advice to help you grow, but with your strong and sometimes inflexible personality, I knew I had to step back and let you learn on your own. However, I want you to know that I'm always here for you if you need anything!

Despite our age gap, the only thing that never changed was supporting one another with sports, achievements and family. Now that you have become more mature, our relationship has been reforged and taken to another level of brotherhood. I'm looking forward to our future not just as brothers, but as men, and to continuing to build our family legacy together!

To Everyone:

I am privileged and thankful for everyone who has been a part of my journey. Not only have you all welcomed me with open arms and love, but you also gave me faith and hope.

Each and every one of you holds a special place in my heart and we've shared many extraordinary moments together. People go through life experiencing challenges and triumphs, and encountering many people along the way. Somewhere along that journey we all realize it is about the village of support we have around us, to celebrate with us in good times and provide support in bad times. I cannot list all the names here, but you are always on my daily thoughts.

I personally would like to give a special thank you to my cousin, Matthew, who has supported me throughout the entire process of writing my memoir. He has worked alongside me as I put my experiences and thoughts in writing, which I hope will inspire everyone who reads it. Without his help, this book might not have come together as well as it has.

I would also like to give a special thank you to Elisha, Dennis, Lian, Elizabeth and Jenn for taking the time to volunteer and proofread this book with their honest feedback and suggestions to make this book spectacular. I'm beyond thankful for all of your help.

Last but not least, I would like to give my sincere appreciation to Lyle and Bobbie Dyment for all of their support of my dreams, for their unwavering friendship and for believing in me. You've both been incredibly good to me and I'm forever grateful.

It's not where you are in life. It's who you have by your side that matters.

To God:

What's the meaning of life?

"To live, to struggle, to serve God."

(An Interview with God)

We all know that you planned for each and every one of us to live for a purpose. Most of us already know what our purpose in life is and others may still be figuring it out. You made me for a specific reason… okay, let's give some credit to my parents too. I am *unique*. There is no one on Earth who is quite like me with my specific gifts, abilities, aptitudes, weaknesses, flaws and strengths. There will never be another like me. I know that, through Your grace, I will strive to be the best version of myself. I will do Your will. One of my strengths in life is that I can show the world that, although life is not perfect, I am able to do Your will and live the life You have planned for me. I trust in You and live with confidence that I am "wonderfully made." (Psalm 139:14)

Introduction

I was inspired to write this book because I want to be a voice for the disabled community, striving to change society's perception of what it means to be disabled. Watching people's facial expressions change when they talk or hearing how they alter their wording to make sure our feelings aren't hurt often comes across as patronizing. We recognize that their intentions are genuine, although it can be a harsh reminder that we're disabled. Quite frankly, none of us will ever need a reminder of our disability.

The purpose of this book is to help show the world that we have feelings and emotions just like you. Our bodies and brains might be different, but we all have dreams and aspirations we hope to achieve. We expect respect and dignity as well as inclusion.

When I look at myself, I do not think or feel that I am lesser than anybody else; I focus on the obstacles I have to overcome. My advice to anyone facing challenges is to assess the situation and attack; knock things down so you can move on. Acknowledge that there will be times when you're faced with the reality of simply not being able to do something. Don't be afraid to reach out and find someone around you who will help you sort things out, give you the honest answer you need to hear or provide the motivation to take that next step. You're only alone if you choose to be. Build that village and enjoy it because you're its mayor. Cerebral palsy changed my life in so many ways, but I'm ultimately in control of my life; I have the steering wheel and I will do my best to navigate the road ahead.

This book is a collection of stories detailing how I've navigated my life thus far. It's filled with memories, memoirs, soul searching, opportunities I was fortunate enough to experience, tributes to those I've lost, frustrations and failures I've faced, and a lot of laughs. This book is my reality and I hope it inspires you to see things a little differently in others and yourself.

Chapter 1:
In a Split Second

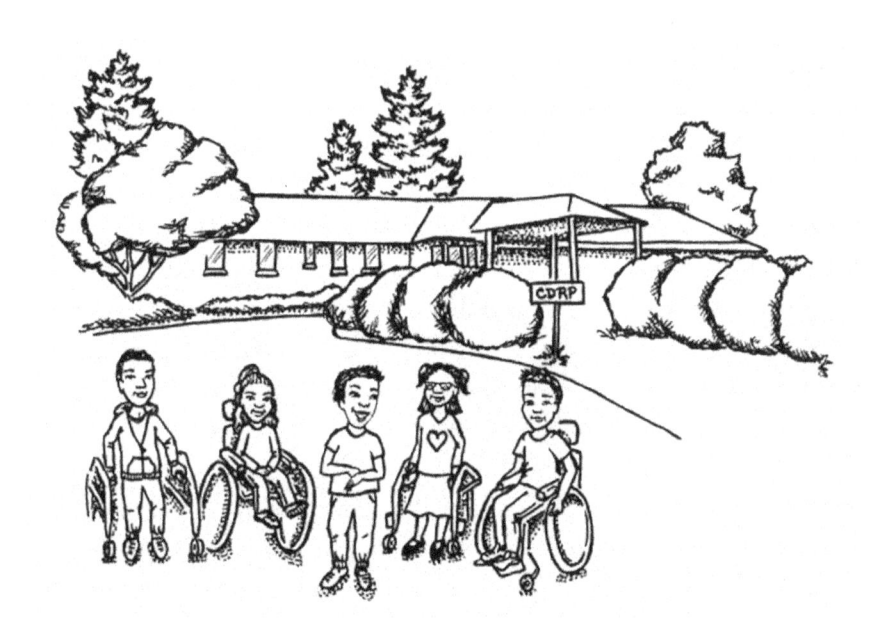

A Newly Minted Scott

On the night of Monday, May 8th, 1989, the family I was about to be born into was enjoying each other's company over roast beef, mashed potatoes and red cabbage salad, or so I'm told. My parents Colin and Silvana Scott were hosting my great-uncle George and aunt Jean for the week as they visited from Florida, with this dinner being their last before heading back down south.

After dinner, my mom began having contractions during her evening bed routine as my uncle and aunt did some last-minute packing. Even though I spent the last nine months enjoying delicious food and the company of friends and family from the comfort of my mom's tummy, I felt like it was finally time to come out to meet everyone in person at that very moment — and maybe I was a little hungry myself and wanted to try some of that roast beef. So, springing into action, surrounded by a mountain of clothes, Uncle George said, "Tonight is the night. I'm taking Silvana to the hospital!"

At 11:00 p.m. that night, my mother started labour. So off they went to St. Joseph's Hospital in Hamilton, Ontario, Canada — *I was on my way.* When entering the labour and delivery unit, my mother was asked when her due date was. The tenth of May was the date that my mother's family doctor verbally gave. The nurse asked for her prenatal papers; these papers have records of the ultrasounds and accurate due dates. These papers, three in total, at different intervals, stated my due date was April 30th. My mother's reply was that "the doctor told me May 10th." The nurse said, "We go by these documents, and all of them listed April 30th as the due date."

My mother was admitted to the delivery unit around midnight after she began experiencing contractions. As the morning progressed, the contractions became closer together, however, she did not dilate rapidly as the contractions were two minutes apart. My father suggested to my mother that she should consider an epidural. The contractions were fairly severe, with only a minute's separation at most times. Given time to think it over, my mother agreed. When my parents took the prenatal class, my mother's labour should have been close to ten centimetres in dilation, with respect to the frequency of her contractions. However, she was only at two-three centimetres and as she felt, the baby was a long way from being ready to be delivered. The epidural was to take the edge off to get some rest for the delivery.

The nurses and doctors were extremely busy with the overflow of babies that were delivered that morning. The nurses were in and out of the room my parents were in to check on my mother's progression. Everything was fine on the fetal monitor at the time. My mother went at 5:00 a.m. to have the epidural. The nurse told my father she will return in a half-hour. My mother was receiving the epidural as the nurses held my mother in a fetal position to get the needle placement and to hold her still. She was experiencing a strong contraction at the time of insertion, so the nurses held her tight. At that moment, my mother felt a crunch inside her stomach and realized her water had broke and mentioned it to the doctor after he had completed the epidural. The doctor more or less said "good" and he left. There was a nurse doing paperwork in the room where my mother was resting and her job was to monitor my mother. The half-hour was up and my mom was brought back to her original room where my father was waiting for her return. The first question my dad asked my mother was, "Is everything okay and what stage are you at?" My mother said that her water had broken and that's all she knows. At that point, she mentioned that she had not been checked by any of the medical team. My father was surprised by that, and just as they talked it over with each other a nurse came in to check the fetal heartbeat and place one on the baby's head. This is when all hell broke loose. The nurse realized that the baby's heartbeat was down to 33 which is very dangerous for the baby. They tried to move my mother around in many different positions, thinking that the umbilical cord could be pinched. However, they put an oxygen mask on my mom's face and took her out to prepare for her emergency C-section.

They had to call in an OB to come and quickly help with my delivery. At this point, I was in distress. Babies that are overdue have a higher risk of meconium aspiration. This means that the first bowel movement a newborn child will have outside the womb, I had inside the womb. I had inhaled this fluid into my lungs causing me to technically begin to suffocate. By 6:00 a.m. I was delivered, but not breathing. I was born with neonatal asphyxia, meaning I was oxygen-deprived long enough to suffer physical harm. In this case, it was my brain that took the hit.

Thank goodness that the OB lived several minutes from St. Joe's. He was awakened by an emergency call from the hospital and they were in need of his expertise for the emergency C-section that was about to perform — *I am thankful to that doctor, he saved my life!* That is how my life changed in that split second.

The doctor explained to my dad that I was in critical condition, appearing blue and not able to take in oxygen. He also mentioned that I had a zero Apgar score, which is a method used to quickly summarize the health of a newborn based on five criteria. The score ranges from zero to seven, seven being normal and healthy.

In talking to the doctor, my dad vividly remembers him saying, "Lightning doesn't strike twice." My dad interpreted this as his way of saying that if I didn't survive, they could try again for another child because this tragic event was unlikely to happen the next time. Angered by the insensitivity of the doctor, my dad told him that it was a matter of perspective and that he wanted the child that was born only moments ago. My dad knew that hope was the one virtue one should never lose.

After the doctor left, my dad gazed out the window, losing himself for a moment, when he noticed a church across the street. At that moment, he prayed for a little mercy: "God, please do not leave me with a child that would be totally incoherent. Please leave me with a child that I can work with. You know how difficult this can be, so please be fair, that's all I ask for."

When my mom returned from surgery, he explained what happened during childbirth and what he had been told since she was heavily sedated during the C-section. He told her that I was stable and on tracheal intubation, and had been taken to McMaster Hospital's neonatal ICU. Three hours later, my mom arrived at McMaster where I was still in grave danger.

The nurses and doctors at McMaster Hospital were very supportive of my parents. My mom has said that the experience there was completely different from the other hospital. "I was so grateful to be there with my son and to receive such wonderful care," my mom says about her experience. "They took control and made our family feel secure because they let us know that we were all in this together and that everything would be just fine."

They put me on a drug that kept me in a paralyzed state to intubate me and make me easier to work with. Being sedated also made sure I didn't use up too much energy fighting the procedure — the energy I would need in the days ahead. I would be in critical danger for the next seventy-two hours.

Two days went by and on Wednesday, I was beginning to show signs of kidney failure, signalling that my organs were beginning to shut down. The next day, I was doing much better and was showing signs of improvement.

I was able to have some breast milk from a bottle that same afternoon. By Saturday, I was released from the neonatal ICU just in time for Mother's Day. What a gift that must have been for my mom!

My mom has told me that everything before and after the delivery happened unbelievably fast. The nurses made her feel rushed and like she was a burden to them. She remembers them saying how busy they were (when wouldn't they be?) and that they would check on her progress when they could. My parents took it as a roundabout way of saying, "Don't bother us if you don't have to." After I was born, my mom was out of it, mostly because of the drugs from the C-section. She was being updated on the situation but had a hard time coming to terms with what she was hearing. She used the word "surreal" to describe the situation as she tried to figure out what she might have done wrong as a mother — what did she do to cause this disaster? "I knew I had to stay focused and positive, and continued to pray for you. You needed me," she has told me.

Concerned for my health, my dad needed some answers. He asked one of the nurses what my future was going to look like. Her response was that I would be a "C student" at best. Again angered by someone's insensitive response to the situation, my dad took that remark and threw it in the trash bin. He wasn't going to take these offhand opinions as gospel, knowing that he would do everything in his power to give his son, finally given the name Kyle Nicholas Scott amid the chaos, the best life had to offer.

My first name was taken from a poem that my great-grandmother Jeannie used to recite to my dad about a lad named Kyle from Scotland. My dad always liked the name so it stuck with him. Speaking of Jeannie, when she met me for the first time, she said she was mesmerized by my big, beautiful, brown eyes. Even though she had dementia at the time, she still recognized the colour brown and the fact that all of her grown children had blue eyes. She must have found it odd to see a relative with a colour other than blue. As for my middle name: Nicholas, was taken from my nonno ("grandfather" in Italian) Nicola D'Agostino.

My grandma Evelyn Scott was prone to giving her family nicknames. When she met me for the first time in the hospital, she called me "Spunky" because I seemed high spirited and brave. She knew that I was fighting for my life and, like a hero from a fairy tale, wasn't going to give up.

When I was cleared to go home by the hospital six days later, the weeks began to fly by. Check-ups at three and six months didn't yield anything significant; in fact, I appeared to be fine, according to the examiners. Things really did seem to be going alright until one fateful afternoon in the backyard. A friendly Mohawk College student, who was studying physiotherapy, was renting a room at my parents' house and would often chat with my parents. The student asked if he could give me an examination that day and noticed that my motor skills were delayed for my age. After gently checking my muscles and range of motion, he concluded that I might have cerebral palsy, a term that had not yet been presented to my parents by any health care professional as a possible explanation for my condition.

When I was sixteen months old, my family was sent to the Children's Developmental Rehabilitation Program (CDRP), where several doctors ran a spasticity clinic. There, doctors told us that I have different tones of spasticity in my muscles. That is to say that I have muscles that are continuously contracted, with major tightness in my arms, hands and legs.

My parents recall the doctor looking them square in the eyes and saying something along the lines of, "Whether you are ready to hear this or not, your son has cerebral palsy." My parents finally had a definitive answer when they left the clinic that day and could seek some much-needed answers to help my physical development. On a separate note, our family doctor assured my parents that my cognitive functions were healthy, so my cognitive development would not be affected by CP.

Knowing that I had CP launched my family into a flurry of programs and appointments. Occupational therapists, physiotherapists and more doctors studying spasticity — each professional assessed what I could and couldn't do, some of which seemed to be more opinion than anything. They said I wouldn't be able to walk, but guess what? I eventually did. I ended up doing nearly everything they said I wouldn't. But in a cruel twist of fate, I actually couldn't do a lot of things they said I should have been able to do. There seems to be a pattern here, which makes me question if anyone knows the full extent of CP. Our guess has been that since I fall under different categories of CP and not just one, it's not a clear-cut case. Most people with CP have more difficulty with either their upper or lower parts of their bodies. I happen to be in between the two. I have better muscle strength in my legs than most, and some parts of my upper body don't function as well as they should. My right arm has a hard time straightening out and has high spasticity at most times. I have learned to control some of it when I am conscious of it. My hands will also curl up and go into deep spasms when I try to feed myself or try any type of fine motor function. These are some of the difficulties that I was experiencing as a young boy, not knowing what was actually happening to me. When you are born with a disability such as mine, did I really know at that time what was normal, how a normal hand can be relaxed, and not going into a tight fist when reaching for something? I had to learn what was normal for you and what was normal for me. I found out very quickly that it was two different worlds.

I started CDRP in 1991 when I was around eighteen months old. This was my first real step in learning to manage my disability. To be eligible for this program, applicants needed to have two physical challenges, which obviously wasn't an issue for me considering how severe my CP is. Five times a week in the afternoons, the staff taught me how to walk with the use of a walker and other implements. The program ended up being great for my mobility and really helped keep my childhood development on track.

Around this time, I gave my parents one of their first laughs. My dad came home from one of his all-day work marathons at the hair salon (both of my parents are hairstylists, which is why I always have great hairstyles). During dinner, he put me on his lap and noticed I was mulling something over in my mind like I was planning to do something. Without warning, I made a fist and punched my dad under his chin, confirming I had a wicked sense of humour.

Finding the Right Fit

I spent the next few years attending CDRP five days a week for half the day during the fall, winter and spring months. It was intense but fun and it helped me tremendously. In the summers, CDRP would stop and I would go for routine occupational therapy and physiotherapy as well as speech therapy. Doctors were keeping track of my progress and kept a close eye on my muscle development.

In 1993, I graduated from CDRP at the age of four. My parents enrolled me in swimming lessons and took me to many different physio programs to help strengthen my upper body and legs. I also went to speech therapy, where I learned from flashcards to give my brain some exercise and to help feel out my cognitive abilities. I also began socializing a lot by meeting other children at parks, family events and play areas.

"We exposed Kyle to all sorts of elements a normal child would experience for their age," my dad says. "He would ride little cars, push kids' walker toys around, and even though he couldn't ride a bike on his own, we still put him on it and safely took him around. He did everything kids his age did. It didn't matter what the obstacle was, he did it."

Around the same time, my parents began searching for an elementary school that would understand my disability and be able to nurture my educational development. Even though that nurse years prior had said I would only be a "C" student, my parents weren't going to take that as being true and made damn sure that the school we were looking for didn't take such a negative attitude toward disabilities.

My parents visited a school where the principal toured them around, eventually bringing them to the special educational department located at the far end of the school in the basement. My parents asked what they would do for me in terms of curriculum and socialization. To sum it up, they were going to keep me in that dull and dismal room, hidden away in a dungeon far from the rest of the student body. My parents walked right out of that school because they could never send me to such a place — *not now, not ever.*

The next school had a lot of stairs. I was still crawling at the time and not walking upright, so it was a safety concern. Then we toured another school that was a big school but my parents said they were put off by the principal's lacklustre personality.

After that, we had the principal of special education from the Catholic school board, who oversaw special education for the board rather than an individual school, tag along with my parents as they proceeded to interview future schools on my behalf. When one school principal realized that a member of the board was part of our entourage, she couldn't have been more accommodating. This principal began showing them around the school with enthusiasm normally saved for the Pope. When my parents left, they both looked at each other and said, "What was that all about?"

The third school we visited was St. Teresa of Avila, which welcomed us with open arms. It was a smaller, one-floor school with well-experienced staff who were eager to take care of all my needs. Impressed by the school's attitude, my parents and I met with all of the department leads at the Catholic board of education. My parents needed to know that it would be a safe environment and that I would receive the best educational resources to support my academic success. Believing the school to be the right fit, I was enrolled at St. Teresa of Avila Catholic Elementary School.

That following September, I began kindergarten with Mrs. Stanaitis. She was a great teacher and she already set a great first impression before the school year when she visited me at the CDRP to learn about my special needs. She was loving, sincere, disciplined and passionate about her students. She actually went to all of her students' grade eight graduations, eventually coming to mine years down the road even though she had long since retired. Talk about devotion.

I was also given a full-time educational assistant named Mrs. Gould who would help me walk, but I mostly crawled on my knees. I had to wear a soft blue helmet to protect my head if I fell or bumped my head into things as I played. For the most part, I was just another kid in the class.

The first few years at St. Teresa of Avila were informative for my teachers, parents and myself. We had loads of time to figure out what tools I needed to succeed in an educational environment. As you read further into the book, I am eternally grateful for the amazing staff, classmates and, of course, my educational assistant Mrs. Gould, who you will read more about later. Even though I was a kid and didn't really understand what life was about, I was able to really enjoy my childhood despite all the hurdles I needed to jump over. I would often ask, "What's wrong with me?" In my mind, I could run, ride a bike and ski like anybody else, but in reality, those things weren't always possible and definitely not something I could achieve without help. But childhood was filled with so much positive energy that it helped me believe I could do anything I put my mind to — and, as you will read, I often do.

That same year, I visited the Moira Institute every day from 9:00 a.m. to 4:00 p.m. for three weeks straight. The name Moira was taken from Greek mythology. The Moiras are the Goddesses of Fate, each one controlling an aspect of the threads of the destiny of man and gods alike. There are three Moiras: Clotho, Lachesis and Atropos, who control the beginning, the middle and the end respectively. It is also said that *Clotho* spins the cloths of destiny, *Lachesis* weaves and measures it, while *Atropos* cuts it.

This was a special program that was offered to me by therapists I was seeing at the time. The program was developed in Hungary and was based on a theory that repetitive motions and movements would allow the brain to find ways to overcome complications from a disability.

Through daily playtime, I was learning to find my centre of gravity and the therapists drilled these exercises into me through repetition. They called it the "One, Two, Three Step." I would take three steps and stand to catch my balance. It slowed down my walking, but it lowered my chance of falling considerably. Shortly after, I started walking on my own after my dad would hold my arm and walk me around to practise. It was like a miracle because nobody knew that I could walk or would be able to and eventually I did.

Two therapists, Margo and Pearl, flew in from Hungary to run this program. Margo had a very, very strong Hungarian accent, and was firm with my dad when it came to understanding the type of CP that I have. She would sternly say, "Kyle has what you call athetoid cerebral palsy." Athetosis is a symptom characterized by slow, involuntary and often convoluted movements of different appendages or extremities. The therapist was absolutely right. She once grabbed my dad's face, held him by the chin and said, "Look at me when I'm going to tell you this because it's very important. Do not let anyone cut his muscles. His muscles work differently than most. They will roll up and never come back down into place if cut. Please promise me you'll listen to what I'm saying." My dad has said that when someone who specializes in a field for twelve years grabs you by the face and makes you promise not to do something, you damn well listen.

In a Split Second

Breaking Out into the World

For those who don't know me, I have always been adventurous. I always looked for new challenges to conquer. I do get spooked out unexpectedly, but who doesn't? It was around this time that I was able to play on a kids' sports team. I loved hockey, so we thought we would give it a try. We knew that I wouldn't have the proper balance to stand on skates and knew I wasn't going to play hockey like everyone else, so we worked with what we had. One weekend, my uncle Tony brought me to an open skate at the Lawfield Arena. He helped me put on regular kid skates and hit the ice. This is one of the fond memories I have of my childhood, but I remember loving the feeling of skating around the rink with my own two feet.

We had just visited Disney World and I wanted a bicycle after coming home from vacation. My parents said they would think about it because they knew how crazy it would be to put me on something that requires good balance. I wouldn't be able to ride the bike independently, but my dad knew I wanted a bike, so he got me one.

After they brought it home, I wanted to take it for a spin outside. My dad used his creativity to enhance the bike to help keep me balanced. He took a cotton belt and wrapped it around my waist and shoulders to keep me as straight as possible. I rode that bike throughout the neighbourhood like nobody else. I would stand up and push the pedals up and down feeling like I was so cool being able to cruise around like all the other kids on the street. My dad stayed beside me the whole time to make sure I didn't have any crashes, which I didn't, but his shins took a beating from the pedals constantly bashing into him. The things parents do for their children.

I am and can be independent. However, like most things in my life, it may take me twice the effort and time to do something that able-bodied people find simple. Some of the more personal things require new ways of going about it. Daily routines can often be so fast-moving that if I were to do it on my own, I wouldn't be able to enjoy the life God gave me. I am truly thankful and blessed to have my parents and everyone else who surround me in my life because they've always provided the care and assistance I've needed to lead a normal life.

Spinal Surgery

When I was nearly five years old, the possibility of spinal surgery was on the table. We were told the surgery would straighten out my back, which would create better posture, and that it was being done on lots of children with CP. The surgeon seemed very excited, believing that this opportunity would be life changing for me and something we would all be eager to pursue.

We knew someone who had had the surgery and it made their condition far worse, and we didn't feel like such a risky surgery was the right call. That poor person who had the surgery couldn't move at all afterwards, so we opted out after meeting with the surgeon who, once again, seemed over-eager to open me up. He reiterated that the surgery was mainly needed to stop my spine from curving abnormally.

Would it have worked out? Would my life be different from what it is today? We will never know, but having someone tamper with the spinal region, which is incredibly risky, wasn't worth the chance to find out. We didn't even bother seeking a second opinion, that's how turned off we were by the idea. However, I often thank Margo for her insight and knowledge regarding my health and well being as well as making us aware of the danger of surgery and its potential negative outcome.

Chapter 2: Starting School

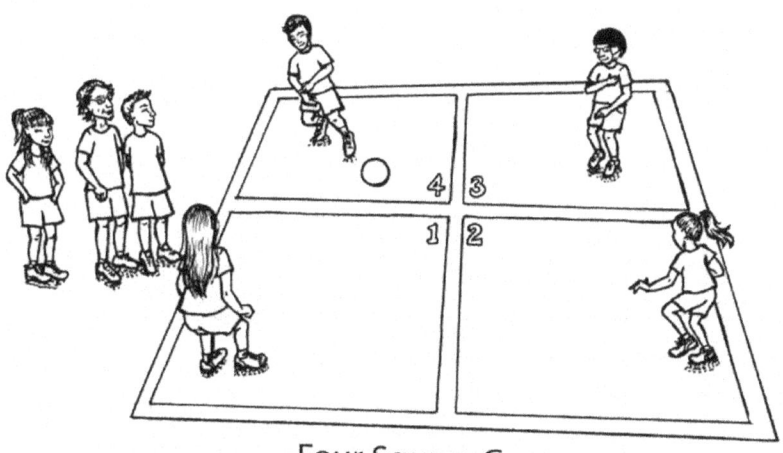

Four Square Game

Continuing CDRP

Between grades one and two, my physiotherapist from CDRP had to figure out which ergonomic chair would best stabilize me in the classroom. In grade one, the physiotherapist suggested a wooden chair that was designed to keep me sitting in an "H" position. This meant that my hips would be at the same height as my knees while sitting properly. My feet had to sit flat on the floor so I could remain comfortable. The seat itself could be raised up and down to achieve the best fit for me.

In grade two, the physiotherapist recommended a kid's office chair for more stability and ease of movement because it also came equipped with wheels. The chair had a red trim with geometric patterns, a grey seat, and a little yellow, red and black accents. It was the most comfortable chair you could ever have to sit in. We jokingly said I finally owned something that would make all the students' mouths water. All of my classmates would secretly have a seat for a minute or two until our teacher was ready to teach us for the day, but the chair was only for me.

Moon-Eyed in Love

When my imagination began to run wild at seven, I got a Playmobil mansion set as a Christmas gift that year. This toy changed my life because at the time I was moon-eyed in love with my first crush named Lauren. She has sandy blonde hair and a mind of her own. She was a little sassy and we hung out a lot during grade one. All of my playtimes changed at that point. I would come home from school and pull out the mansion where Lauren lived. A little Playmobil person acting as me would arrive at her doorstep and swoon when she opened the door. We would take our time kissing in each and every room of that house. I would propose to her and on the same day, we would have a wedding ceremony and drive off in our magical Playmobil carriage. I would guess that we got married about five hundred times before I was over it. If those toys are still kicking around, I'm sure they're still married today, penniless from the weddings, but probably happy all the same.

Meeting My Best Wombat

Grade one was when I met a boy named James, who I'm very close with to this day, but it wasn't until grade four that we started hanging out with each other. We would play every sport you could think of during our after-school hangouts. The two of us would also partner up for class projects whenever we got the chance. One of the earlier projects we worked on had a special meaning for us that we still reference today. James and I were assigned a geography project where we had to pick an animal to study. We chose an Australian animal called the wombat.

If you don't know what a wombat is, it's a short-legged, muscular, quadrupedal marsupial that is native to Australia. Wombats have a cute face but look like a weird combination of chipmunk, squirrel and bear. They're about the size of a small dog, with stubby tails, and they can weigh up to seventy-seven pounds. They mainly hang out in forested and mountainous locales.

We had a blast learning about this cute and funny-looking animal. This is when we began calling each other "Wombats." James insisted on being Wombat Senior, which made me Wombat Junior, even though I am older. To this day, we still use these nicknames for each other as you will read in the stories throughout the book.

"This Is My... Tent Party"

My birthdays were different every year. In 1999, we decided to camp out overnight in a tent in the backyard. We had a BBQ just before dusk settled in and then we went to our tents to watch movies. It was a nice temperature for May.

However, the night did get a little crisp. We had a ton of snacks so there was a lot of plastic crinkling and food crunching happening. The one thing that stood out from that night was the divide in the movie selection. Some of us liked the options while others didn't. Robert, a friend and classmate at the time, wanted to watch the horror movie *The Evil Dead*. It's not uncommon for boys to pick scary movies during sleepovers, but James was terrified and went into the house to help my mom clean up so he would have a reason to not watch the movie. That little wombat still hates horror movies to this day.

The divide between the fearful and the confident was all too apparent at this point. Robert had nerves of steel at the time, or at least it seemed that way. As for the rest of us, well, it took some time for us to build up our manly demeanours. We ended up watching *The Evil Dead* followed by *Sister Act*, of all movies. James didn't stick around, but we soldiered on without him. We all came back together the next morning for some pancakes and bacon despite the thrilling evening in the wilderness.

Laws of Gravity

In grade seven, both my class and the grade eights went on a school trip to Ottawa, Ontario. After an early start and six long hours on a bus that morning, we finally made it for a class tour of the Supreme Court of Canada building in Ottawa. We were running a few minutes late and my dad, my teacher Mr. Mauro and I had to take another way into the building because it wasn't wheelchair accessible. Can you believe that? Needless to say, we were scrambling so we wouldn't miss anything.

While in transit, my front wheel got caught on a slightly lifted curb and since I've never worn a seatbelt while in my chair, I was sent flying through the air. Thankfully, I was able to walk it off with my own two feet with help from Mr. Mauro, who grabbed onto the back of my t-shirt. Unfortunately, my dad wasn't as lucky as he got his legs caught between the wheels trying to save me. He had a few cuts and scrapes, but we both came out with no major injuries other than to our pride.

The next morning, we were having completely different difficulties, but not with me this time — *instead with my friend Ryan*. He simply wasn't getting out of bed. Mr. Mauro knocked on their door in the hotel and my best friend James answered while he was brushing his beautiful white teeth. James said, "Mr. Mauro, we have been trying to get Ryan up for the last half-hour and he is not getting up." Mr. Mauro immediately went into the room and all we could hear from a few rooms over was, "Ryan, get up! Let's get moving!" repeated over and over. I'm surprised the hotel didn't come storming up to our rooms.

Finally, Ryan slowly began to turn over, gave a big stretch and yawn along with a sound that I could only describe as an animal being slaughtered. I remember Mr. Mauro laughed and said something along the lines of, "Ryan. That's the ugliest face I have ever seen in my life! Let's go!" before we finally got on with our day.

Starting School

Relentless Practical Jokes in Canada's Comedy Capital

Before the summer of 2003, both the grade sevens and my grade eight class did a few church tours while on our school trip to Québec. The first location was the Saint Joseph's Oratory of Mount Royal, which is a Roman Catholic minor basilica and national shrine in Montreal, Québec. Its claim to fame is being the largest church in Canada and it has one of the largest domes in the world.

This class was filled with incredibly inconsiderate students. As an example, when I was getting on the bus, they would push themselves through the front door of the bus, shoving me into the wall, albeit gently. To get back at them, my dad and I decided to play tricks on them by saying, "Is that a five-dollar bill on the ground there?" or "Is that a mouse under the bus?" When we did that, getting on the bus was easy because everyone was too busy looking around for invisible money.

When everyone settled themselves down, we took a peaceful ride into the forest to Érablière le Chemin du Roy, located ten minutes away from downtown Québec City. We experienced a warm atmosphere in the forest that could play host to any sort of celebration imaginable. Very picturesque and magical. Érablière le Chemin du Roy stands out because of its beautiful setting and excellent food.

We learned about the 300-year history of maple syrup and how it's made from scratch. Our homeroom teacher, Mrs. Pimenta, and French teacher, Madame Mattina, had us form a circle for a sing-along. We also grabbed our "magical spoons" that we brought with us. Magical spoons are a musical instrument made out of wood that resemble two spoons connected together at the handles' end. If you've ever seen someone playing the spoons on their leg, it's pretty much the same concept.

While everyone was outside getting fresh air and looking around before heading back inside the cabin, my dad pointed at this big, dark thing moving through the forest. He described it as a black horse. The special education teacher, Mrs. Brady, who was with us at the time, had a puzzled look on her face. "My God! It's a black bear!" my dad yelled with unwavering conviction. I could see the panic on Mrs. Brady's face and decided to egg the situation on by yelling, "Run into the barn for cover!" She would have fallen for it if it hadn't been for someone else nearby confirming that it was just a black horse walking around. It was almost the perfect practical joke and would have had an amazing payoff if it had worked.

The next day, back at the hotel after another day of touring about, the teachers and other students wanted to get back at my dad for all the jokes he had played during the trip. My dad can be relentless sometimes so it's completely understandable.

My dad went to the lobby to use a telephone to call my mom. When he returned, I was "nowhere to be found" and he proceeded to go from room to room asking everyone if they had seen me. A few of the teachers also played along by pretending to look for me as my classmates and Mr. Mauro moved me from room to room to stay out of sight. My dad looked all over, fearing that I might have fallen somewhere. He looked behind a vending machine and in different rooms, and then he thought he would visit the students I mostly hung around. There I was, hidden away in one of their rooms. My dad said it was, "Game on," and laughed it off with all of us knowing that he wasn't going to take this lying down.

While in Québec, we also visited the Canadian Children's Museum. Ryan asked my dad to hang onto his wallet because his shorts didn't have any pockets. After our visit to the museum, we gathered on the bus to take it back to the hotel. Ryan takes his seat but has a look of sheer panic on his face. He was feeling his pockets, tossing his backpack around and searching the seat next to him. He finally shouted out, "I have lost my wallet!" He asked around if anyone spotted it, but nobody had. Ryan looked so sad as he sat down defeated. My dad, not wanting to pass up yet another opportunity to yank someone's chain, asked Ryan if he was absolutely sure that he had lost the wallet and hadn't given it to someone to hold for him. Ryan was sure he had it on him all day. My dad pulled the wallet from his pocket and presented it to him. "Where did you find it?" Ryan said with a wave of relief appearing on his face.

As we were touring Old Town Québec City, we came across a cool landmark that was a tree called the Tall Old Elm Tree. The tree, located on Rue Saint-Louis at the corner of Rue du Corps-de-Garde, has a large cannonball trapped in its gnarly roots. Although there is no marker to indicate how the cannonball got there, the rumour is that it became lodged during the war of 1759 between the British and French and the tree just grew around it. It's a unique yet iconic landmark in Québec City. I thought this was such a neat landmark to see.

Later that evening, we walked through the beautiful park in Old Town Québec. My classmates would take turns pushing me in my wheelchair. James was excited to help out and after enjoying the smooth ride with my new "driver," I found myself travelling a little too fast and realized that I was about to be in serious danger. Remember, I never put my seatbelt on in that thing, which I was about to pay for dearly. The next thing I knew, James was turning me around a tight corner with incredible speed and while my body weight was shifted to the left side, KABANG! Both of us ended up mangled on the ground. Thankfully, it left me lying on the ground and not six feet under it, only leaving a few grass stains and an incredible sense of stupidity.

I loved both the Ottawa and Québec trips because of the level of independence I had. The amount of social interaction I got to experience with my classmates was so much fun. It was like a dream come true at the time.

Reflecting on My First Ten Years of Life

During my early years, I was quite busy with school, occupational therapy, speech therapy, physiotherapy and sports. Things able-bodied people can do were things I had to work at. I had daily assistance with personal duties and feeding — not because I was unable to do it for myself, but because it took and still takes me twice the time or longer. As I grew up, I was able to be much more independent until my hip dysplasia kicked in later in life, which took away some of my independence.

When things fell into place, I was living a life just like every other "normal" kid. I did well with my education, had amazing classmates, made friends and enjoyed just being a boy. But did any of that keep my mind off having CP because my life was busy? You might be surprised, but I would say it absolutely did.

For the first five years of my life, I was only able to crawl on my knees or when someone held both of my hands to walk a few or more steps, as you do with infants. After going to the Moira Institute for three weeks, I learned how to walk on my own. Can you believe that? Three weeks! Once I got home from the program, I would practise with my dad until I was able to walk on my own two feet. It felt so good to be able to walk and run independently. I walked at home and at school, but I used my manual wheelchair for longer distances like at the mall, on school trips, walks/hikes and going to the park. The only thing that was frustrating was the inability to write and draw. My muscle tone wouldn't allow me to have the control other people have. I specifically had this issue with my right hand.

I remember in grade three, I was sitting at a table with classmates who were drawing things. I wanted to join in, so I grabbed a pencil and paper for myself and started to draw a face on a body. When Mrs. Gould came back to the classroom after her break and saw what I had drawn, it shocked her because it was actually pretty good for someone in my situation. Obviously, my spasticity made it difficult to draw anything, but I managed to pull out something resembling a face. Everybody was so proud and amazed that I was able to draw, so much so that everyone wanted their own copy. As time went on, technology advanced and I began typing and "drawing" on a computer. Having a computer was a big help moving forward because I was able to get tools that helped make it easier for me. As technology progressed, I soon became equal with my peers in the skills that they used to communicate on a daily basis. Who would have thought that writing was going to be replaced by a keyboard.

After overcoming many obstacles during those years, I received the "Yes I Can Award" in elementary school for the poems I wrote. The award is given to students with disabilities who overcome challenges that were initially difficult for them to perform. If a student worked hard and diligently all year and successfully achieved their goals, they would be recognized and given the award. There was even a dinner to honour all of the students who received one. Families, educational assistants and teachers would come to the event in celebration of the award recipients.

There were actually two events each year for award winners: one was at Michelangelo's Banquet Hall and another was a sports activity day. The sporting event was held at the Lieutenant Governor's Invitational Games in Toronto, which played host to a variety of games. One of the games was floor hockey and since I loved playing in net, I hopped in it when I was given the chance. One of the photographers took a ton of photos that day, which I barely noticed, but you know that saying, "the right place at the right time"? Well, the photographer captured a picture of me making a big save during the game. I didn't know about the picture until my uncle Mike called us a few days later to let us know that I was on the front page of the *Toronto Sun* newspaper. Seeing myself there made me feel like a young Special Olympics athlete.

I always participated in everything my classmates were doing during recess. We played some entertaining sports like basketball, soccer, ball hockey and four square. I was exposing myself to new challenges and working on staying upright as much as I could. My walking was always jerky looking, but I could still move around on my own two feet and that's what mattered.

In my later years of elementary school, I remember walking out into the schoolyard and being able to turn around on my own to see my shadow. Normally I needed assistance, but to be able to do it on my own while walking gave me a sense of pride. I think that kind of illustrates the progress I made and the challenges I overcame as a kid, you know? It was the simple things most people don't even think about that I had to work at. It was a struggle, but I was determined and didn't give up on myself.

Graduating Grade Eight

The class I was in from junior kindergarten through to grade eight was hailed as the best class during those years. All of us were told this many times by our teachers, supply teachers and other staff who watched us grow up.

While not everyone was kind all of the time, for the most part, my classmates in those elementary years at St. Teresa of Avila were friendly, and many were close friends.

My classmates Carolyn and Carla were the sweetest, prettiest and most helpful friends that anyone could have as a kid. Carolyn was always the one who would look out for me to make sure I always had what I needed. Every day for half an hour when Mrs. Gould was on her lunch, Carolyn would sit with me after recess to take notes for me and that was a deed no one could take away from her. She thoroughly enjoyed helping out. Carolyn and I received a Christian Attitude Award in grade eight because of our relationship and behaviour that year. We remain good friends to this day.

Carla was always kind and caring, and treated everyone equally, which isn't an easy thing for a kid to do. Carla was always ready to help with anything I needed. She would replace and sometimes steal some of the duties Carolyn took pride in. I still keep in touch with both of them after all these years.

Our grade eight graduation was boat-cruise themed — you know, as in "bon voyage," have a good trip. We spent most of our time during the last couple of weeks before grad making this piece of a ship with big rolls of manila paper in the gym. It felt like we were legitimately building the Titanic with all the work we were putting into this thing that would set sail for only one night. All of us drew or at least attempted to draw our adorable faces in each of the portholes along the ship, so you can imagine how terrifying or, maybe, awesome that must have looked.

I was so excited about starting my next chapter in life. Although the thought of attending high school was exhilarating and nerve-wracking at the same time, I was emotional knowing that I had to part ways with my educational assistant, Mrs. Gould, who had been with me nearly every day for ten years. I always found it comforting to have someone watching out for me during those years. Here's what she had to say about that day.

"I felt both happy and sad that day," recalls Mrs. Gould. "I was happy to know that Kyle was a dedicated and hard-working student. He was always happy and eager to learn, and he worked so hard to get to where he was on that last day. It also made me happy to see his parents so pleased to see how much he had grown and progressed with their support and guidance. We were very lucky to have such a wonderful class; everyone genuinely cared about Kyle and included him in all school activities. I was happy to know that everyone involved in Kyle's learning and development did their very best to help him get to that day. However, I was sad because I was retiring in the fall, and I knew I wouldn't have the pleasure to see Kyle and his classmates grow into the fine young adults they are today."

Starting School

After the grad ceremony at our parish, Regina Mundi Catholic Church, we made our way to the gym for our celebration. The first dance was the mother-son and father-daughter dance. As I was dancing with my mom, we both looked over and realized Mrs. Gould was bawling her eyes out and, of course, tears began rolling down our faces too. My heart broke because I knew exactly how she felt. Over the past decade, she helped build me into the person I am today. The bond that we shared and the level of communication we had, with all the laughs and growing pains, made her like a second mom to me. So I knew what she was feeling and we all shared happy tears together for a moment.

My dad took both of us outside to calm down where we realized that my dress shirt was soaked right through from crying. I changed into another dress shirt that we brought with us and went back in for more dancing. When I returned, Carla and I danced together during the first dance before everyone was allowed to join in and it's a moment that I will cherish for the rest of my life. The rest of the evening was filled with more sad goodbyes and best wishes as everyone reminisced about the past ten years we had spent growing up together. What a milestone to graduate grade eight.

Reflecting on those years, I am extremely grateful that I had the best teachers who taught with passion, believed in me and pushed me to be the best I could be. I thank all of them for making me "smarter."

My classmates... well, I couldn't have asked for more amazing group to share the journey with. We all shared lots of great memories, some of which you've already read, during those ten years. From the bottom of my heart, I thank each and every one of them for not only accepting me for who I am and believing in me, but also for always for including me in every activity and the games we played at recess, especially when we discovered the most favourite and entertaining game called *Four Square* with the only rule exception being that I could use my legs and feet. All of them always helped when I needed a hand, especially when I was laying on the ground after falling. I also won't forget the many times they fought one another over who was going to pick me up. It was truly an honour to feel so looked after.

I am very fortunate that I have had an educational assistant like Mrs. Gould for ten straight years. Not only did she support me with my education, but she also helped build my confidence and self-esteem. Such an incredible gift to have been given.

I will never forget how the principal of my school actually tried to take Mrs. Gould away from me quite a few times. He felt that we were too bonded and close. My parents were floored by such a ridiculous reason. The principal eventually elaborated by saying that students who reach puberty should be paired with an assistant of the same gender. Well, that only lasted a week because educationally I was far beyond what the new guy was capable of handling. I was once again paired with Mrs. Gould from that day forward and we shared many wonderful memories. She retired at the end of 2003, not long after I went to high school. We're still in close contact and remain friends to this day.

Chapter 3: High School Life

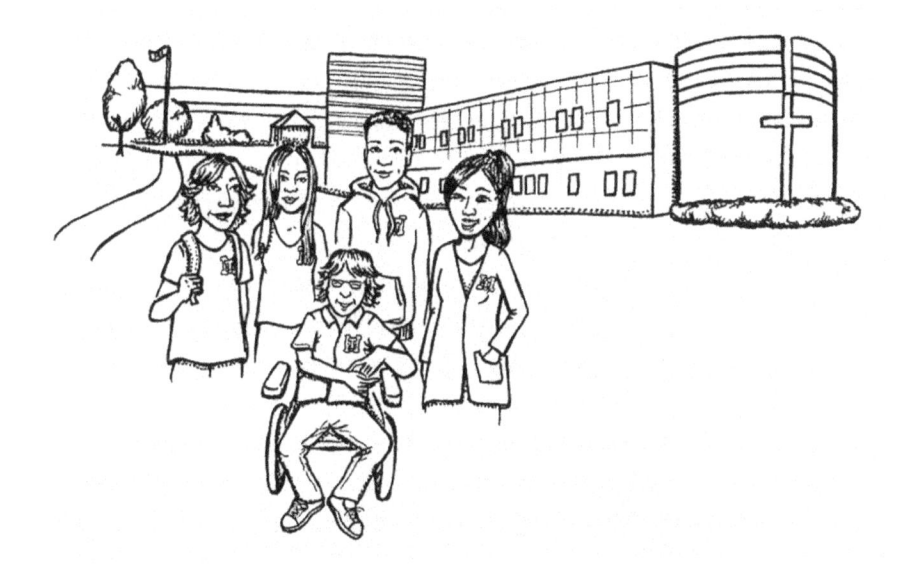

The Shy High School Guy

The summer ended and I entered a whole new chapter in my life: high school. I attended St. Thomas More Catholic Secondary School. In the beginning, I was a quiet person. I spent most of the time in the Special Education (Spec Ed) room because I didn't even know anybody yet excepts my classmates from elementary school, but we all had different timetables and courses.

I was very self-conscious about going to the bathroom because I wasn't comfortable by just having someone help me that I didn't know yet. There was an instance where my dad took me to the bathroom (during my lunch on the first Monday of the school year) in the Spec Ed room and when I came out, the head of Spec Ed, Mrs. Gera, asked my dad what he was doing in the students bathroom. She didn't recognize my dad, so thankfully that was defused as fast as it had arisen — otherwise, it would have got messy. But it ended up happening a few times more anyway. Mrs. Gera claimed it was because my dad and I don't look a lot alike at first glance and they thought he might have been my wheelchair sales rep. Well, he did show the staff how to use my chair in manual mode if the battery ran low this one time, so I guess that kind of makes sense. We all had a good laugh at the bizarre situation when it was all said and done.

During my lunch hours, the Spec Ed department wanted me to have lunch in the cafeteria with other students. With there being three periods, a lot of my friends were scattered all over the place, whether still in class, somewhere else in the school or out getting lunch. I spent a few of my lunches with a male educational assistant (EA), who wasn't a good match for me. I mentioned this to Mrs. Gera and she switched me to another EA, Mrs. Langille, who worked with me a few times in grade eight while I attended St. Teresa of Avila.

Mrs. Langille would accompany me during lunch and we talked about a wide variety of topics, like my hopes of having a girlfriend, going on dates, always being a part of social engagement and among my peers, that sort of thing. She definitely got her exercise each day because we would travel around the school for a good chunk of the lunch hour.

There was a school dance each month at the school, but the first month was only for grade "niners." At first, I was too nervous to go and decided I wouldn't bother. Mrs. Clement, who was one of the special education resource teachers (SERT) at the school, asked me if I was planning on going to the dance. I told her no, but she insisted that I should go for my first one just to see. I thought what the heck, it could be fun, so I ended up going.

Thankfully my cousin Alisa, who used to babysit my brother and me, was one of the prefects at the school. She was supervising the dance so I made sure to take her as my wing-woman. An entire bench filled with my friends showed up as well, so I ended up having a great time after all. The next time I saw Mrs. Clement at the school, I thanked her for convincing me to go and I ended up going to quite a few dances throughout my high school years because of that first experience. Like I said, I was very shy at the beginning. I was out of my element and felt like I had to start from scratch again.

By the end of that semester, I had EAs fighting to work with me though. When we were getting ready for exams, Mrs. Gera created a large paperboard with all the special needs students' classes and teachers for the next semester. The EAs had to sign their names beside students they wanted to work with. Mrs. Gera had the final say, but when she was trying to make the final decision for the pairings, she called me into the office. "You're making this hard for me," she said. I asked why and she told me that all the EAs were fighting to get me as their student. I was pleasantly surprised at first but eventually said, "Wow, I must be special."

Pow, Pow, Power Wheels

In the early days of high school, I was forced into having a laptop strapped to my wheelchair so I could use a program to convert text to speech. This would help me communicate with others as they adjusted to my speech. I absolutely loathed it and fought to have it taken off. I never felt more uncomfortable driving around with a laptop and huge speakers attached like a mobile radio station. We had several meetings with the Technology Access Clinic (TAC) to try to find a better solution.

The occupational therapist (OT) from the TAC aggressively denied my request to leave class a few minutes early to save myself the embarrassment of being seen in this contraption. The OT said I would use that time to impress everyone with my laptop and would just socialize instead of getting to my next class. Mrs. Gera and I looked at each other and laughed, knowing how bullshit that claim was.

Mrs. Gera scoffed and said, "Kyle, you should definitely do that with two thousand students rushing to get to their next class with only three minutes to make it. Cute girls can fall into your lap and you say, 'Hello, my name is Kyle.'" Navigating around all those students after each period with open lockers, bags on the floor, students fighting or whatever else teenagers do in three minutes was hell. It was impossible to see where I was going since I was lower to the ground and, honestly, it made me feel claustrophobic at times. But yeah, let me put on a show for a minute to impress my peers while all this is happening. All of my teachers ended up letting class out a few minutes early anyway so I wouldn't be stuck jammed in the hallways. They even told the OT at some point and made sure to point out her lack of compassion toward my needs.

Golf, Leafs, Golf

In grade nine, the last period of the day was religion with Mr. Curtis. He was a Boston Bruins fan and had a teddy bear with a Bruins jersey on his desk. The second he found out I was a Toronto Maple Leafs fan, we started teasing each other every single day.

That year, the Leafs were knocked out of the playoffs before the Bruins were. Mr. Curtis would remind me every time I saw him that my boys were out golfing while his team was making their way toward the Stanley Cup. I would always tell him not to worry because the Bruins would be joining the Leafs on the course soon enough.

Shortly after the Bruins were knocked out of the playoffs, my best friend James, our classmates and I wanted to tease the heck out of Mr. Curtis. So, we took his teddy bear and taped the arms so it looked like it was crying. When Mr. Curtis entered the class, he saw his Bruins bear shedding imaginary tears. He immediately looked directly at me like I did it. I pretended to swing a golf club and said, "A nice day to tee off, isn't it?"

Later that year, I discovered how small this world really is! After showing my yearbook to uncle Tony, he noticed that I had been taught by one of his former teachers, Mr. Curtis. My uncle was excited that he could connect with him again through me. We had to come up with a scheme to play a trick on Mr. Curtis, so I brought him a can of Pepsi which was his favourite beverage. Mr. Curtis had no idea what was going to happen to him in the hallway when I asked to speak to him.

I handed him a can of Pepsi, he looked at it and said, "How did you know this is my favourite drink?"

"It's from a D'Agostino," I replied. "Tony as a matter of fact."

He could not believe this, he remembered my uncle of course, and said, "Well, yeah... you guys do look alike." It was a trip down memory lane for Mr. Curtis that day, as he quenched his thirst at the same time.

Patience and Respect

Even though I knew that my OT and Mrs. Gera were trying to give me the best possible devices to help me at school, I would still rebel against using them. A few stories back, for instance, I wrote about the laptop and speakers that were attached to my wheelchair that helped with my communication issues. When I felt like these devices were unnecessary, of course, I would push back. I know my limits and I like to prove people wrong. I don't want to give up before I've even had a chance to try for myself.

I know my articulation isn't always clear, but I've found that once people take the time to speak with me, they begin to understand what I'm saying. It's not perfect, but all I need is for people to focus, listen and treat me with patience and respect. I don't want to be written off because of my disability. I realize that we as people with disabilities, need some support in the sense of communication. Equipment that is available to us has given those who cannot speak a voice. This voice allows us to express ourselves in many ways, breaking down those walls of silence. In my situation, I work so hard on my vocabulary in order to articulate the best I can. I didn't want to ever loose that ability and solely depend on the voice recognition program. I just hope that people will support and continue to encourage as much verbal conversation with me, and whomever wants to use their words.

My educational assistant, Mrs. Stevens, was persistently told to ensure I used my devices. She knew I loathed them and would tell my OT and Mrs. Gera that she could understand me just fine without them. I only used the equipment when I was either forced to or just to please others, until I managed to finally win the battle right before first semester of grade ten ended. All this equipment would constantly get smashed and bashed by students, staff, walls, doors, pretty much anything that existed around me. I eventually won that battle and only used the laptop in grades eleven and twelve for AutoCAD. As time went on, everyone started understanding me, so I didn't need to bother taking the time to type everything out constantly. We could finally have normal conversations instead of sitting through long pauses while I was typing a response. It definitely made for better conversation.

Given No Slack

Back in grade eight, Mrs. Gera had a meeting with me to see where my education level was. She didn't fully believe that the academic level of my work was of all my personal input. Her thoughts were how much of my work was supported by the EA, meaning, were they doing all the work for me. They soon realized that I did meet the full potential of the academic work that was assigned to me and more.

During grade ten, Mrs. Gera, felt like I wasn't reaching my full potential. She paired me with a younger EA named Mrs. Cino just in my civics and career classes. The idea was that Mrs. Cino would whip me into shape somehow.

We had a rough start, to say the least. I felt like she was pressuring me. After a few days of working together, I spoke with Mrs. Gera privately about how I felt. I explained that Mrs. Cino was giving me a hard time by pushing for detailed answers to questions. I would give an answer, Mrs. Cino would write it down and would respond, "More details!" Mrs. Gera said she knew this already because she instructed her to not let me slack. She also went on to say that she wasn't about to let four years of school blow by without seeing what I had to offer.

I got what she was saying and once I understood that, I respected both Mrs. Gera and Mrs. Cino even more. We managed to work out our differences and get on the same page as we moved forward and I was better for it.

Turnabout is Fair Play

"You will either love me or hate me," was the first thing my grade ten civics teacher, Mr. Luvisa, told us in our first class with him. He was a stickler for start times since the class was at 8:20 a.m. If you weren't there on time, you were locked out like a fool until the daily announcements were over. Sometimes he would let you into the class if you were late depending on the day, but not usually.

Like they say, "turnabout is fair play." One morning, everyone was in the classroom except Mr. Luvisa. The announcements came on the TV and there was Mr. Luvisa doing them. I looked at Mrs. Cino and asked, "Should I lock Mr. Luvisa out?" with my mischievous smile. She didn't give me a verbal answer but instead flipped the power switch on my wheelchair to give her approval.

The door shook as Mr. Luvisa tried to open the door. He was peering in through the little window in the door asking to be let in while laughing. "Kyle, I never thought I had to worry about you," he belted out. Ah, the sweet and delicious icing of revenge.

Prom Night

I was excited to go to my prom in November 2005. I had hoped to have a girlfriend or, at least, have the opportunity to ask a girl by this time, but it didn't work out. Originally, I wasn't intending to go because I didn't have a date, but I didn't want to feel sorry for myself and it wasn't like I would be alone with so many friends around.

The first order of business: getting to Carmen's Banquet Centre where the prom was being held. Easier said than done when you drive a power wheelchair. Unfortunately, we did not have an accessible power wheelchair van so we engineered two planks of wood to create a ramp to get my wheelchair in. Not the safest idea, but I can jokingly say I've driven the plank.

At every social event, students had to be checked by security for any alcohol or drugs or weapons or who knows what. As I was in the lobby area waiting for all of my friends to come in, one of my SERT teachers, Mr. Sartor, told me that I needed to go through security. I've always been known as a goody two-shoes and he saw this as a golden opportunity to try to sabotage my reputation. I was confused because I had already been there for at least an hour and asked him why. There was no winning that argument, so to the back of the line I went.

As a quick side note: Mr. Sartor and I have an interesting connection that I found out during high school. He used to coach my uncle Tony in football while he was in high school. Tony actually played for the Hamilton Tiger-Cats. He was drafted in the sixth round, forty-fourth pick after playing for the McMaster Marauders for four years. After finding that out, Mr. Sartor and I formed a jovial relationship with him, nicknaming me the "Twenty-buck Man" in reference to always being surrounded by girls.

Now, where was I? Oh right, prom night... back in the security line, a guard checked behind my power wheelchair and found a plastic bag. I wasn't worried because I knew it wasn't mine. The guard rummaged around and found something. With a shocked look on his face, he pulls out a few bottles of rum and schnapps. Out came the handcuffs and I was read my rights. I was a little shocked, to be honest, but I had a feeling I was being pranked. I looked around for the culprit and I locked eyes with Mr. Sartor for a good laugh. The whole thing was staged as Mr. Sartor made sure everyone was in on it from the beginning. It paid off and was completely worth it in the end.

Besides nearly being arrested, the rest of the evening was a blast. I had a great dinner and danced with all of my friends, namely the girls. I still had some obstacles I needed to overcome that night; one was being stuck in a wheelchair. How exactly can you dance with someone who's standing when you're sitting? It was awkward but we all made it work. The second was spending the night at a hotel with friends. I couldn't do it and I still lacked the freedom I so desperately wanted in my life. Instead, I watched my friends get a nice evening away from their parents.

In order for me to attend these types of overnight events, I need someone there to look over me. Think about how you would feel having your parents around listening to all your conversations. Think about being around your friends, but your parents have to escort you to the bathroom when you need to go. It has nothing to do with love and respect for my parents; it's about personal space. Don't all kids want to be free from their parents' rules? I think it's only natural.

Despite my apprehension, I am glad I went to the prom and thankful for the people I got to celebrate it with.

High School Life

People Watcher

In grade twelve, my last class of the day was physical education. One of the SERT teachers, Mr. Mombourquette and my guidance teacher decided to look for a peer helper to help me with any activities during gym class.

They found this nice and easygoing guy named John. We knew each other through mutual friends, often exchanging pleasantries in the halls as we passed by each other. I've always been a people watcher, so I'm pretty good at guessing people's personalities by observing them. I had a feeling John was a really good guy and would make a good friend. So, it's funny that now we've been brought together and finally have a chance to know each other.

After a few weeks of John helping me out in class, we instantly became good friends and he introduced me to some of his friends, including this guy named Blake who shared my passion for hockey. We had a blast doing workouts, running on the treadmill and using the exercise bike together. Sports were a lot of fun, too, and I've always been grateful to have a buddy there for me when I needed one during gym class.

Graduation Year and Applying to College

Grade twelve was my favourite grade in high school by far, although by the end of it, we were all super excited to graduate and head into the next chapter of our lives. I had grown so much over the past four years, really coming into my own and becoming more comfortable with myself and those around me. I was a real social butterfly, striking up conversations with everyone, (especially with the girls). My friends could always find me at my favourite location in the school, which my physical education teacher referred to as "The Speedy Parking Spot." The spot was just outside of the Phys Ed office and had clear views of each end of the hall so I could see people coming.

One of the nicknames I picked up over the years was "Moses" because when I drove through the hallway people scurried to the sides of the hall to let me pass as if I were parting the Red Sea. The funny part was this often happened in the religion portion of the school, where a painting depicting the Crossing of the Red Sea was prominently on display. You either followed me to get around faster or jumped out of the way so as to not get your foot run over.

Each day for four years brought new challenges, goals, dreams and adventures. I'm really proud of myself to have been on the honour roll for my entire high school career. I shared so many memories with my peers. Some were good, like all the fun and laughs, while others were sad and heartbreaking. From grade nine to twelve we lived and experienced, we matured and grew with knowledge. That's how we all found ourselves in the end before heading off to our post secondary educations.

On our Graduation Day held at Hamilton Place in downtown Hamilton, we were the first graduating class to have over four hundred students graduating at the same time. It was a great honour and I was proud to take the stage with my fellow students. When it was my turn to wheel onto the stage in my power chair, my EA, Mr. Friend noticed I was nervous and gave me some words of encouragement by saying, "Whatever you do, don't run over the bishop." I came out to an enormous roar of applause and clapping. I made it to the middle of the stage before my hand began to spasm. I thought for sure that the bishop was a goner, but I managed to regain control of myself before reaching him. Praise be to the Lord, no one was run over and it all worked out great.

One of my classmates who had been in my English and Religion classes, Sylvie, snuck up behind me within seconds after our three hour long ceremony was over and gave me an unexpected kiss.

Because the actual graduation was a monster event, we had our graduation dinner and dance the next night at Liuna Station, again in downtown Hamilton near the Bayfront Park. The entire evening was a blast and the memories will last a lifetime. I echo the words of my friend John who gave a speech as a class valedictorian during the ceremony: "To my fellow Knights, goodbye my friends. God bless you all!"

Reflecting on all those years made me realize how much I had to go through just to make it through. It was overwhelming entering high school and wasn't made any easier when I had to go through testing so the school could collect some data on my aptitude. As I've mentioned, it was stated quite early by the school that my grade eight work wasn't my own. I'm glad the testing clarified that mess, but just imagine having to prove your competence and abilities to enter post-secondary. They did put me in a few general-level classes, like math, that I eventually moved out of because my work was far more advanced. My math teacher even spoke up to signal that I needed to move up to the advanced class. I really did have a lot of great memories from high school that I still cherish today and won't forget everyone who helped me along the way.

To my educational assistants who worked with me during my four years at St. Thomas More (STM) high school, I cannot thank you enough for all the hard work you all put in supporting my education and being a useful right hand, unlike my own. Not only did we share moments on an educational level, but we also shared many conversations and laughs together throughout the years. I think we covered the whole world in terms of the topics we spoke about.

To Mrs. Gera: The first time we met during your visit to my elementary school, you were having a difficult time believing that some of the work I was completing was mine. You thought I didn't take school seriously and just wanted to have fun. I knew I had to prove my capabilities to you and it was something I knew I was ready for. I was proud to be given the chance to prove to you just how capable I was and I was overjoyed when one day you told me, "Kyle, you have proven me wrong, you are an intelligent young man. You have earned my respect." Mrs. Gera, thank you again for believing in me, pushing me to reach my potential and basically kicking my butt!

To the late Mr. DeMarco: Thank you for supporting my education and looking out for my best interests. We shared many laughs and secret jokes together during my last two years at STM. May you rest in peace.

To all of the teachers who supported me in my education, it was a pleasure being in all of your classes. Thank you for all the tools you gave me to apply toward my secondary education. We shared many laughs and teachable moments together.

To my fellow classmates: The four years of high school were the best four years of my life. I have heard that many kids generally don't have a great high school experience because they didn't fit in, they may have been bullied or went through awkward/rough patches in development. Except for an adjustment period I experienced in grade nine, I was very fortunate that everyone I met accepted me for who I was and made sure I was doing okay. Thank you to everyone who made an impact on my life.

The Three and a Half Obstacles

High school was the best four years of my life. Sure, the first semester of grade nine was spent adjusting, facing challenges and having butterflies in my stomach, but didn't everyone feel that way? However, as time went on, everyone got to know me and I was able to be myself. I guess you can say I came out of the bubble I was in.

Once I was more comfortable, I began venturing out of the resource room to meet new friends. Thankfully, my cousin Alisa, EAs, staff and teachers encouraged and pushed me to experience what it meant to be a high school student. I really am grateful for that.

Even though I was a well-known, sociable and lovable guy who got involved in many activities that were going on, I still feel like I missed out. I definitely wouldn't change a thing that I've done, but I would never get past the three and a half obstacles I needed to face during my four years in high school.

The first was wanting to be in a relationship. I still remember how badly I wanted a girlfriend. I had asked a dozen girls out, if not more, whom I was interested in dating. There was no doubt that they liked my personality and enjoyed hanging out with me, but they only wanted to be friends. Honestly, this was always heartbreaking for me because I felt like I didn't deserve to have a girlfriend because of my CP and might not have done enough to make someone interested. I felt like it was my fault for something I didn't have control over. Even though I beat myself up over it, it never changed or stopped me from being who I am as a human being. I understand that being a teenager is difficult at most times when it comes to confidence and peer pressure. I knew that I didn't stand alone with some of my feelings. I could look around and see my peers, hearing them expressing their heartfelt feelings, knowing that they felt just like I did. I knew then that I was not alone in this awkward stage of my life.

High School Life

I have an extreme passion for playing sports, but having to find ways to do it my way becomes my second obstacle. It was extremely difficult not being able to play on any of the high school teams for obvious reasons. Deep down I knew I would have contributed all of my passion, sportsmanship and leadership to the team. Even though I wasn't physically on the team, I was with them in spirit and attended games to cheer them on. My good friends James, Ben, Ryan, John and Blake all played on different sports teams, but there I was supporting them in the stands. I also went to girls' basketball, hockey and volleyball games of course — *I'm not stupid!*

I remember when St. Thomas More won the Ontario Federation of School Athletic Association (OFSAA) Football Championship. They won the first back-to-back senior football championship, which was a huge achievement in the school's history. The school also won many other OFSAA championships.

I couldn't have been happier watching what my friends accomplished athletically. My long-time friend, James, won championships with the boys' basketball team with Ben and Ryan. Unfortunately, Ryan decided to transfer to Bishop Tonnos the following school year. It was a new high school and had smaller class sizes — *what a traitor, eh?* James also ran OFSAA cross-country each year and won the Athlete of The Year in grade ten. John was part of that back-to-back OFSAA championship victory with the senior football team. He received a defensive MVP award for his hard work. Blake was the captain of the boys' hockey team. And of course, my brother Stirling with all his games I attended to show my "brotherly love" support. I was extremely proud of all of them. As you can see how I reached out to be a part of the team, not the part of playing with them, but supporting and cheering them on. That helped fill the void in my life, feeling I was right there beside them every move they made.

As I've mentioned, it was extremely difficult to sit on the sidelines and not actually play on high school sports teams. Sledge hockey eliminated that pressure and disappointment because it gave me freedom. It more than made up for what I felt was missing in my life and helped me cope with feeling left out. It made me feel like I could challenge myself physically and be part of something bigger. I loved meeting new people and sharing a common interest and passion in something so many people rallied around, and I'm beyond grateful and privileged to have been a sledge hockey player.

However, I was grateful and had the privilege of managing the St. Thomas More girls' softball team. One of the SERT teachers and coaches, Mr. Mombourquette, knew how much I loved sports, not to mention girls. He asked me to help run the team with him, telling me that he wanted to inspire the girls. This wasn't a difficult decision to make.

Mr. Mombourquette came up with the phrase, "Whenever you're on base, come back home to Kyle," to encourage the girls. I truly enjoyed helping out with the team and felt honoured. If you're reading this, thank you Mr. Mombourquette and Mrs. Clement for that opportunity!

Attending and supporting all of my friends in their sports made me feel like I was part of their journey. That feeling really helped me overcome that obstacle of being left out and not being able to physically participate.

The third obstacle was wanting to be independent and free of help. When you're a teenager, you want to hang out with your friends as much as possible. Unfortunately, I struggled with privacy and independence for the first two and a half years of high school.

This was around the same time when I found out that I had hip dysplasia. Most people didn't and still don't realize how much pain I was in, but I also hid my emotions because I didn't want it to take anything away from me, plus I'm not one to complain. However, bedtime was a nightmare for months on end. It took me twenty to thirty minutes just to get my right leg straight and comfortable in bed.

After a few years, my hip found a spot where it could rest peacefully and the pain decreased considerably, nothing like what I was experiencing in the past. This spontaneous miracle gave me my life back and allowed me to walk again. My walk was still compromised as my gait was off and I needed to rebuild the muscles needed to walk, but I could get up again and that was all that mattered to me.

I started going to the YWCA for a workout program run by CDRP to get those muscles going again. After a while, I was getting the hang of it again, but nobody at school knew I could actually walk because they had never seen me do so. One day, I got Mr. Friend to stand near me in case I fell and just got right up to walk around. I scared the crap out of the department heads, EAs and everyone else who was there at the time. I remember Mr. DeMarco yelling, "He's healed!" as I lumbered about.

Boy, did it ever feel good to be able to stand on my own two feet and walk around again. So when I had gym class with Mr. Friend and my peer helper John, I was at the top of the world again. When I was able to participate with my classmates running and doing laps, it felt good to be able to experience that. Mr. Friend and John had to run with me, each holding me up under my arms as we ran around. Are you picturing this? It made me feel stronger and more able to handle challenges that would come my way.

From there, I was able to do a lot more. For the first time since grade eight, I was able to play a little ball hockey. It only lasted five minutes before I lost my balance and went knee first to the floor. Poor John felt so bad because he was unable to catch me in time. I made sure he didn't feel too guilty and assured him that this would happen all the time back in grade school.

Being able to move around on my feet brought me a lot of joy. However, it was still an obstacle for me when I couldn't go to Blue Mountain Resort with my friends over Christmas break (for those who never heard of Blue Mountain, it's a skiing resort). Most of my friends went and I felt like I was missing out. Thankfully, I had great friends who kept me involved during their trip so I could somewhat experience it through them.

It had been a few years since I was able to go to house parties, but I was finally strong enough to walk independently. John, Blake and the rest of the group hosted parties that led to great memories of us socializing, drinking beer, watching sports and playing cards. I was so happy to experience those things with my high school friends.

Now you are probably wondering what "The Half" obstacle is. At sixteen, most teenagers get their driver's licence. However, this didn't affect me as much, because I knew that driving would never be an option. Not only did I not want to be in danger, but I didn't want to put anyone else in danger, either. I remember my civics teacher, Mr. Luvisa, asking me if I was going to get my driver's licence. I laughed when he asked and told him, "I already have it. How do you think I'm driving this power wheelchair?"

I know for darn sure, and given the fact that I have spasticity, I would probably be swerving all over the road. There's no doubt that days exist where I would love to jump into a vehicle and just drive anywhere I wanted. I would also have a nice, vibrant, lime-green car that would catch everyone's eye as it's my signature colour.

According to most people, I was actually not a bad driver, especially going into the SERT office where I had to navigate desks, chairs, boxes and staff members just to have friendly conversations with Mrs. Gera, Mr. Mombourquette and others.

Chapter 4: College Years

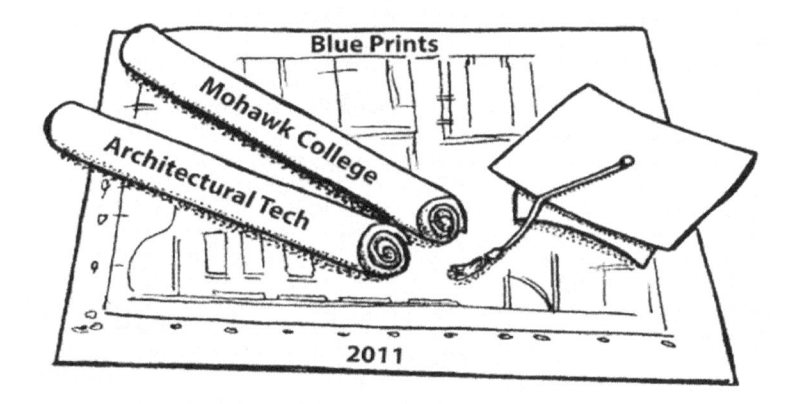

College Acceptance

While in high school, I was being advised to stay until I was twenty-one to help prepare me for college. I didn't want to waste my time there even if I was nervous about taking that next step in my education. I also didn't want to get left behind by my graduating class as most of them went off to post-secondary; this was an opportunity to do what everyone else was doing. The head of the special needs department at St. Thomas More jokingly said that I was either crazy going to college so young or just a brave soul ready for his next adventure. And that's what this was to me, a new adventure and a place to make new friends and develop a career.

I applied to the Pre-Technology course at Mohawk College in Hamilton with the goal of getting into the architectural design course. I didn't apply to other schools because Mohawk was close to my home and was known for having a great program. I was accepted, which got me very excited because I knew I was following my heart. We met with Mohawk to make sure I would have the proper support in place during my post-secondary education.

I started school the following semester, but I needed to upgrade my math while there, so I spent that first year getting everything I needed from the pre-tech course while upgrading. The next year, I jumped into the architectural design course with both wheels. I've had no regrets going through the program because I've always had a passion for design and being able to see a project come to life. I think this is a genetic thing because a lot of relatives on my mom's side are engineers, architects or some kind of designer.

First Day at College

My first day at Mohawk College was exciting, but I was nervous. Once I found out there was another student with CP named Justin who was taking Pre-Technology with me, it really calmed my nerves and we became fast friends. He actually joined my sledge hockey team that year as well. Between college and hockey, we spent a lot of time together; sometimes seven straight days together. It got to the point where we would see each other and have a look of "Ugh, you again?" on our faces.

Justin used a manual wheelchair because he was strong enough to push himself around. There was a very steep ramp at Mohawk's front entrance that everyone would have difficulty with. I would always ask Justin if he wanted to hop onto my chair or get a tow up the ramp. He would hang on to the handle of my powered wheelchair as I took him. We would also do this if we had classes at opposite ends or floors of the school. Sometimes, I would crank up the speed, so when I did a quick turn he would crash into the wall.

Between classes, we would grab snacks. Justin would sometimes help me eat things, like a double chocolate doughnut that would end up all over my face if my EA or personal support worker wasn't there. At the end of the day, we would race each other on the same steep ramp toward the DARTS bus to see who could catch more speed.

One of my courses was split between Drafting and AutoCAD. Drafting class was where I learned how to draft manually on a drafting board. Because of my CP, my hand doesn't have the strength to write let alone draw what's called a construction line. My spasticity put an end to that pretty quickly because, as you can imagine, a defining characteristic of a line is its straightness. But if you want squiggles and scribbles, I'm your man.

My class instructor, Elizabeth, and I found ways to allow me to participate in the class and how my grading would work. The second part of the class, which was AutoCAD and computer based, was where I really shone. You need to be able to manually draw blueprints, which isn't something I can do. So instead, I had to study and learn how to read them. However, I ended up acing the AutoCAD tests because I can do everything everyone else can do on a computer. It helped that my teacher always made sure that I understood what it meant to have a keen attention to detail.

Overall, my first semester at Mohawk was fun and I learned a lot. I ended up doing very well in all of my courses, including Drafting and AutoCAD, with an overall grade of 100 percent. I also made the Dean's Honour List, which is always something to be proud of.

First Year of College Done

After my first full year of Architectural Technology, and failing Surveying in the first term and Estimating in the second term, my coordinator of the program suggested that I switch to the technician program, so I could focus on something less intense.

That first year was very involved and I had to always find ways to overcome my physical challenges. For instance, I had to hold a survey lens, look through it while standing and be completely still. Obviously, that doesn't work at all for me because of my spasticity. When I was in class trying to apply theory while navigating a surveying camera, I found that I was missing out on major information that you can only get if you're capable of performing the task manually.

I repeated that course in the summertime, bringing all the things I learned previously with me. Having taken the course before really helped me to better understand what needed to be done and I ended up getting marks in the high 80s. I didn't give up. I just had to work out what I could and couldn't do physically and to work around the logistics of it all. I had to mesh my skills and abilities together and learn new strategies, but I did it my own way.

My Last Years as A Student

College came and went just like that. I had lots of challenges to overcome, but I overcame them. I didn't let my disability prevent me from getting a diploma. I didn't have many expectations going into college, but it far exceeded what I thought college would be like. It wouldn't have been possible without the students and friends I met, the instructors, the EAs and all the support staff who were incredible. As a group, they were all very supportive, encouraging and good company.

Once again, it was time for me to spread my wings and fly. This time, I was faced with entering the real world, which smacked me right in the face. No more school, just the reality of having to get a job.

The graduation ceremony was long but great. We all went backstage dressed in black robes. I noted the feeling this time around compared to my grade twelve graduation. Everyone seemed calm and relieved to graduate instead of being nervous and anxious. I felt like it was the weight of all the hard work and stress being lifted off our shoulders, and knowing that we could finally apply what we had learned to future endeavours. Students still cheered and caused a ruckus, but there was a maturity to it.

Thank you to all my Mohawk College instructors who inspired me to be the best architectural technician I can be. Some of you have said that I was one of your most inspiring students that you've taught in your years, which made me feel fuzzy inside. However, I couldn't have done it without all the tools that you provided to me.

To Alyson: I remember the first time meeting you. You were the exam supervisor for one of the exams I was doing and my EA was unavailable.

For some reason, I immediately felt a connection with you and wanted you to work with me for the rest of my time at Mohawk.

When I was having some issues with my original EAs during that time, whom both left at the end of the first semester. I went to the disability services department and requested you. I was so happy you agreed to work with me.

From the day we started working together to the day I graduated, we worked well together, shared lots of laughs and built a wonderful friendship that remains today. Thank you for supporting me all those years.

To Carmen and Joan: Both of you were my education lifesavers when Alyson was unavailable to come in for the day. Not only were we able to get some work done or take notes during the lectures, but we also shared many laughs together.

Thank you again for everything you have done, making the effort to substitute for Alyson and being my saviours. I am so thankful we've remained friends today.

Being Disabled and Work Don't Mix

Since the day I became an architectural technician, and earning my AutoCAD Design Certificate in 2011, I applied to jobs every day. Growing up, I always had a passion for designs and looking at houses, which was why I chose to become an architectural technician, hoping to bring designs and ideas to the table.

After a year of Pre-Technology, I had a meeting with the chair/associate dean of the building and construction sciences (BCS) department at Mohawk College to discuss my goals and future in this industry. The dean said, "Our instructors will accommodate your needs and I'm sure you will get good grades. However, I am more concerned about working in the workplace because of the situation you are in." I didn't take it as discrimination; the dean was being upfront and truthful.

Over the years, I have applied to tons of jobs posted on Indeed. I had my resume professionally proofread by the Mohawk College jobs centre. One of the employment consultants suggested not mentioning my disability on the resume because it would prevent me from being contacted by employers and I totally agreed. However, receiving phone calls is another obstacle that I have to face. I can speak over the phone if that person knows me, but my articulation may not be clear when I'm nervous.

When I got phone calls, my parents had to speak on my behalf, which is a little humiliating. I know if I weren't in the situation I'm in, I would be speaking myself. Once my parents explained my situation to the person, then the "red flag" went up. Some were very understanding and others were brusque, such as:

- "I expect his work to be like others."
- "I will speak it over with my boss." They called a few days later: "Sorry, we will not be moving forward with Kyle."
- "Sorry, we are looking for someone who can do multiple duties, including taking phone calls and going to the job sites."

In 2018, I finally found an employment agency for people with disabilities. They would speak to the person I applied to and advocate for me. More recently, some companies are now contacting you through emails. One day, I received an email from one of the jobs I applied to stating that they wanted to set up an interview. I got my agency to call them and go through things about me; the guy said, "I'm not interested in moving forward with Kyle."

During these years, I tried going another route besides just applying to jobs that were posted. I would personally send an email explaining my situation and what I had to offer. They were all quite impressed with my designs and pleased with the fact I had reached out networking. I even self-taught designing pools and turning someone's backyard into an oasis — I created YouTube videos of my designs as well. However, it still didn't get me far.

While I am extremely proud of my educational accomplishments, I find it both humbling and sometimes humiliating as I have remained in the same position, looking for employment since graduating from college.

Looking for Work

I began looking for work after officially being an architectural technician for only a month. My dad had a client at his salon getting his hair cut who was a teacher at my old elementary school, St. Teresa of Avila. He graciously mentioned my situation to an architect who was working on a project for the school at the time. The architect was kind enough to sit down with me to go over options for future employment and to act as a sounding board.

We set a meeting at his office and went through a bunch of different options I could pursue. He said he was impressed by my portfolio and that might have been the only words of encouragement he gave me. His basic suggestions were to start at the bottom, keep up with current design trends and to sell myself. "If you have to sweep the floors, you sweep the floors," he told me. I don't know if he got the impression that I was looking to start at the top or was gunning for his job, but it's pretty obvious that you start from the bottom.

He mentioned that I should do volunteer work, reminding me yet again that you have to start from the bottom. I said that volunteering is a great opportunity to get some experience and your foot in the door if you can get someone to take you on. So I asked him if I could volunteer for him, but he turned me down stating that he "didn't have time to oversee something like that." See what I have to deal with? The Hamilton area doesn't have an abundance of architects and most of the ones that are around aren't wheelchair accessible, which I learned trying to hand out resumes. Imagine that, an architect not thinking about the accessibility of their buildings.

In September, a client at my dad's salon was saying that her grade eleven daughter was looking for a co-op placement with an architecture company. My dad interviewed his client while he cut her hair only to find out that the girl had landed a position with the same architect whom I had met with months earlier. A student with little to no skill goes over me, someone who graduated with honours and knows the industry-standard design programs inside out.

That man I met several weeks earlier had sat there and told me a hard-knock story of what to expect as I looked for work in my industry only to take a chance on someone with no experience. He knew I would have jumped at an opportunity to get my feet wet. I guess he wasn't seeing me for me and was too busy looking at the wheels attached to my hips.

First Job Interview in Person

After years of applying and phone calls, I finally got a job interview with a renovation company about fifteen minutes away from where I lived. I was really nervous since I didn't have much interview experience, but it went very well. My verbal articulation was a little off because of my nervousness, but we managed to get through it. The owner was very impressed with my portfolio and skill set, asking how I was able to design everything that was in it. I felt a sense of respect from him I don't normally get from people.

A few weeks later, I received an email from him that stated, "Thank you for applying and coming in for the interview. Unfortunately, we have decided to go in another direction. Best of luck in your future."

Despite striking out, I felt a sense of accomplishment because I got a callback and that proves there is interest in my expertise. I got the impression that if I had been the right fit for the job, I most likely would have landed that position. It just wasn't meant to be that time around.

Life Is Expensive

As you know, life is expensive, but think about my life for a second. How can I provide for the lifestyle I want to lead? I receive money from the Ontario Disability Support Program (ODSP), but that's peanuts and certainly not enough to cover what's needed for me, let alone what's needed for a basic family household. ODSP is a great system for people with disabilities and I'm grateful for the service that's provided, but it truly isn't enough.

In my world, I need full assistance to complete routine tasks. I need to be fed, helped in the bathroom and clothed every morning. Think of the overhead I need for care, then add on utilities, rent/mortgage, a cell phone bill, Internet, food, etc. I need those things, especially a phone and the Internet because it really opens the world up for me in terms of communication and entertainment. If you add all those things up, you'll see that ODSP doesn't cover it all. I've tried to make a living off my talents and trade, but without a steady paycheque and opportunity to make a living, I haven't been able to make that extra money on top of ODSP needed to survive. I would like to have enough money to enjoy a social life at the end of the day, but none of that seems possible in my situation.

So again, the question remains: how can I provide?

Chapter 5: My Sporting Career

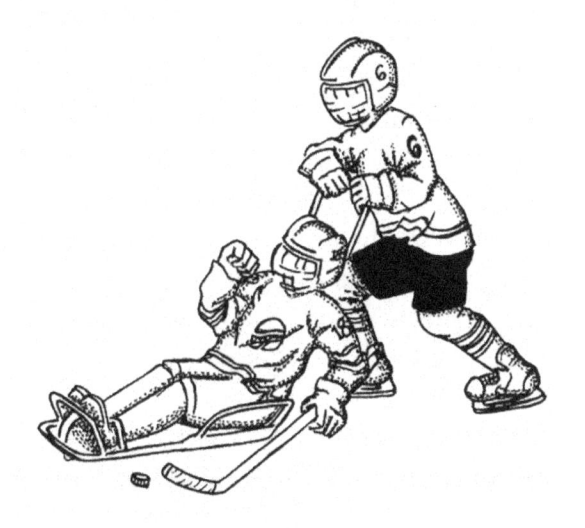

In this chapter of my sporting career, I have written some of my memories from my years in sports. I hope I can inspire someone to get involved in a sport that you have a passion for and create your own memorable sports stories.

As I've mentioned earlier in the book, one of the things that was extremely difficult was not being able to participate in high school or extracurricular sports teams. However, I was very fortunate to be born around the time the community created athletic opportunities for those living with disabilities. I was four years old when I started playing with the Hamilton Challenger Baseball Association and six years old when I started playing with the Hamilton District Sledge Hockey Association. I met wonderful players with natural athletic ability playing both as teammates and respectful adversaries.

An Unexpected Dive

On Saturday, August 11th, 2000, I had an opportunity to play on the Hamilton Challenger all-star team for the Challenger Baseball Tournament in Oshawa.

My first time at bat, I made a good hit that soared straight down the middle to centre field. As I was running toward first base, I was also keeping an eye on the ball to see if I had enough time to make it to second. And I did! I decided to take the risk and run to second base. Just about five feet from the base, out of the corner of my eye I realized that the ball was speeding toward my destination when I was nearly there. The only choice I had was to take a dive for it; otherwise, I would have been called out for sure. My helmet came spiralling off as I hit the dirt and it rolled a good few feet away from me. My body made contact with the base, so I knew that I had made it. My spotter, a volunteer who ran with me in case I needed help, hoisted me back to my feet and I immediately looked at the umpire to see if I was safe. The suspense was killing me because I didn't normally do something so risky, but sure enough, I was.

A lot of people thought I lost my balance by tripping over my own feet, not thinking it was intentional. That's totally understandable given the obvious circumstances, but I surprised them with my play.

I was thankful for the opportunity to play in the tournament and to the Hamilton Challenger Association for choosing me to represent the all-star team that year.

Jealousy on the Ice

In 1996, at the age of six, I started playing sledge hockey at the Chedoke Twin Pad arena in Hamilton, Ontario. I was unable to push myself around. My uncle Tony would take me to practice on Saturdays and be my pusher. The sledge looks like a toboggan with skates and has a handle out the back

My Sporting Career

like a stroller for someone to push. I only had the use of my left arm, so I would hold the stick in my left hand and play the game just like anyone else. My uncle pushed me for a few years until he started a family of his own, welcoming his first child and a new cousin for me, Samantha.

In October 2000, sledge hockey season came quickly and it was the first year that I was able to play on a junior team, which meant travelling to different cities for away games. I had my first-ever away game in Stratford, Ontario, at the William Allman Memorial Arena, which was built in 1924. Surrounded by history, I felt like I was in an NHL arena.

The team got on the ice to warm up for the game. Our coaches called everyone to the bench to tell us the line-ups and game plan. One of my teammates couldn't stop his sledge while coming toward the bend. He ended up sliding right into the back of my dad's skates, which sent my dad flying backwards on the ice. Everyone, including the people in the stands, saw my dad airborne for only a second and collectively let out a gasp as he slammed onto the ice. He landed on his back and, luckily, didn't hit his head, so he collected himself, got back up on his skates and turned to the stands shouting, "I'm alive! I'm alive!" Thankfully he wasn't hurt at all and we were able to continue the game.

During the game, a Stratford player twice the size of me was receiving a pass from his teammate near our net. I quickly made my way over to him and put my stick under his arm and pushed him into our goalie knowing that the referee wouldn't be able to see me hooking the player. Bang! Right into our goalie, we went knocking everyone down. My devious plan worked out because the referee gave the Stratford player a penalty for goal-tending interference.

This was the year I became friends with a girl named Christy who has been a client at my dad's hair salon since she was a little girl. In the summer of 2000, my dad asked Christy if she would be willing to push me in sledge hockey that coming fall. Since my dad knew she was a special service worker and loved being active, he thought Christy would be a great match to help me get around on the ice. We spent some time getting to know each other over the summer. We were fairly aggressive toward one another, always teasing each other, with me often telling her that she couldn't keep up with me. To this day, I keep reminding her that she still can't.

53

When we finally got on the ice for the first time that year, I thought, "Wow, she's awesome, I love her." She's full of enthusiasm, passion for hockey, soccer, ringette and was a Schiehallion Dancer to boot. Obviously, a cute young energetic blonde girl was what I wanted — *on the ice*. Christy would run us into the boards, checking other players against them as we fought for the puck. Christy would always tell me to throw my body into players who were chasing the puck and to dig for it. "If the referees had a problem with it, they could take a hike," she would say with conviction.

The season continued and our biggest rivalry was with the team from Mississauga. It wasn't because we were neighbouring cities, but because I had a pusher. Both teams were very aggressive toward one another, even toward Christy. What drew me to sledge hockey was the fact that I could have someone safely help me participate, and the game itself is host to many people with all sorts of challenges. However, Mississauga only took players who could push themselves, and even worse than some of the players were the parents.

At one of the games, my mom overheard an aunt from the Mississauga team proclaim, "That kid with the pusher would never be allowed to play on the team if he couldn't push himself!" Instantly furious, my mom marched right up to her and asked what her problem was. The lady turned around and repeated what she had just said as if nobody around her heard her the first time. "That's my son you're talking about and he loves playing hockey," my mom scolded. "This game is for anyone — it's not the Olympics!" The woman didn't like hearing that one bit, but everyone around her had to educate her on the rules and sportsmanship of sledge hockey.

Sometimes during games with Mississauga, I would get a penalty for going too fast. Yes, you read that right. *Going. Too. Fast.* In hockey. Have you ever heard of such a thing? The word on the rink was that the refs were told to keep on my pusher during their games to give them an edge. Sounds like absurd jealousy to me and they shouldn't have taken themselves so seriously. Their team had a lot of fast players and you can bet your skates that they were the same ones having their egos hurt. They were notoriously dirty players.

There was an instance where one of the Mississauga players grabbed my stick and held onto it. I threw my hands up in the air, while the guy still held my stick, and yelled at the ref to draw attention to it. No penalty was given. Not even so much as an acknowledgement. That's pretty pathetic and proves that there was favouritism happening. Despite all this nonsense, Christy and I ended up having a great season that year, scoring at least one point per game, but it goes to show you that anything can be ruined by selfish behaviour.

As Blind as a Baseball Bat

I was a competitive baseball player and known for base-stealing when I played, but there was one instance I might have been a little too into the game. My uncle Brian was pitching for my team and while I was up at bat, I made a good hit that soared straight down the middle of the second and third bases. As I was running to first base, somehow I threw my bat over the fence. The umpire told me that if I did that again, I would be ejected from the game. I apologized and told him that it slipped out of my hands, but he didn't believe me and stormed off.

The following game, the same guy was umpiring the game. I was at bat again and hit the ball to third base. I ran to first base and in case you needed a reminder, I have CP so my balance is off at the best of times but I knew something else was wrong here. In my head, I thought that I had made it to the base just a split second before the first baseman caught the ball. However, the umpire called me out. Okay, fine, this guy clearly needed his eyes checked, not only because I should have been safe, but also because first base wasn't correctly lined up on the diamond.

I walked back to the bench annoyed, but the other team's coach, Ron, saw how disgruntled I was and came over. I told him about the base being off the alignment and together with the "blind" umpire, we examined it. We walked in a straight line from home plate to first base to discover that the line was off by about a foot. Turned out I was right in the end, but the call had been made and we made the discovery after the inning finished, so I was out anyway. Justice wasn't served that day.

By the end of this season, I knew it was probably the last time I was going to play any sport independently. I had been playing sports since I was four years old with my dad, Uncle Tony and a few others supporting me along the way. The previous November, I found out that I had hip dysplasia (having a hip joint that would often dislocate, due to the deterioration of the hip and the ball joint). This answered why I was beginning to have so much difficulty walking and in pain. Some days I could walk, other days I needed a wheelchair to get around. There was no way I was going to play in a wheelchair, so I decided to retire. I wish it could have lasted longer, but some people don't have a chance to play at all. I am grateful to have had the opportunity to play baseball for ten years and enjoyed every moment of it.

Driving Through a Blizzard

Without fail, every year when we would travel to London, Ontario, for the yearly Invitational Sledge Hockey Tournament, there would be heavy snow. For the 2005 tournament, the weather decided to play a practical joke by dropping a blizzard on us, and I'm not kidding, the team is called London Blizzard. Only my dad and I made it up for this event because my mom had to take my brother to his own hockey games.

My poor dad had been dealing with kidney stones since Christmas, so he was often in severe pain. We were about twenty minutes away from the event location before we started running out of windshield washer fluid. Between the snow and the road salt, we couldn't see a thing. We followed the blue flashing light of an emergency vehicle to get off the highway to refill. We managed to pull into someone's driveway and the owner actually came out to offer assistance. My dad told him we were all good and would be on our way in the next minute or two. Then it hit him... another kidney stone attack.

I could barely hear my dad moaning in pain inside the car but it was written all over his snow-covered face. I saw him turn away from the car to relieve himself at the side of the road. "Tomorrow that guy is going to think I murdered someone because I finally passed that stone," my dad said when he hopped back into the van. As we sped out of there, I could see blood sprayed all over the snowbank where my dad went pee. I can only imagine how painful that must have been and what the homeowner's reaction would be when he found the crime scene.

We managed to get to the tournament, only missing half of the first period and with us already losing 2-0. I quickly got dressed and hit the ice. I helped the team tie the game up with two assists before it ended in a draw. The next day, we played two more games. We lost 5-2 to Elmvale and tied Kitchener with no goals from either team. We managed to do well but we were just a half a point short from moving on to the quarter-final. We were all very proud of our performance that year but were disappointed that we didn't make it since we finally had a good team put together. For some of us, including me, it was our last tournament at the junior level. We celebrated one last time together by going to East Side Mario's for dinner, after which I returned to the arena to watch the final games.

While I was looking at the standings posted on a wall, Coach Peter, who coaches one of Hamilton's intermediate teams, introduced himself and asked me if I was planning on playing the following year. Yes, of course, I was going to play, but had to ask him if having a pusher could pose an issue. It turned out that it wasn't an issue and he told me how much he appreciated my hockey IQ.

That following summer, I started practising with the intermediate team named the Hamilton "Bar-Ken" Sledgehammers since there were two intermediate teams from the same city. Everyone there welcomed me with open arms, making me feel like I had been playing with them for years. My former pusher, Christy returned home after graduating from Brock University in St. Catharines after a few years. Nothing has changed besides getting older and, maybe, wiser. I was up to my old tricks again, teasing and disagreeing with things just to annoy her. I would sometimes pick a fight with her in public to give the appearance that she was beating on a disabled person.

This was the beginning of a whole new chapter in my sledge hockey career. A rookie reaching for new experiences and goals — and a new haircut, not by choice. The entire team hazed me into shaving the beautiful, long curly hair I had at the time. I led them on for a bit and they thought they had me, but they backed off because they knew how attached I was to my hair. Not only that, they knew that if I chopped it down to the woodwork, I would be the most handsome guy on the team and they would be jealous.

Coaches Doug and Peter had six rules to follow while on the team:
1. Have fun.
2. Within reason, give each and every player an equal amount of ice time.
3. Teach each other the basic, new and advanced skills with the objective of improving your own skills over the entire season.
4. Always be aware of every player's health issues and never compromise their safety.
5. Be competitive while playing within the rules of the game.
6. Keep all players' family members informed and involved to the extent of their ability and interest.

The Second Coming of the Dynamic Duo

Christy was like a big sister to me and we always had each other's backs. A lot of the teams we played against did not like us much because we didn't follow the "pusher rule." The rule states that a pusher cannot go faster than the slowest player on the ice. The rule was often abused and we both knew people would pretend to be the slowest just to get us caught. Then when we went off the ice, the opposing team would suddenly start flying around the ice with newfound speed. Christy was very vocal about the obvious abuse and pointed it out to the ref who would just tell us to slow down. "Not a chance in hell," Christy would say under her breath. It's obvious why I like her so much.

After a couple of months as a rookie intermediate player, I earned my coach's trust by improving my skills to the point of becoming one of the top two liners. Being in the top lines is a privilege bestowed to players who have proven themselves over time. When I first started out, I was playing on the fourth line — the last line. Over the span of three months, I worked my way up to the first and second lines.

The more aggressive our game was, the more aggressive Christy and I were. When we were on the bench, getting some fluid in, Christy said, "The faster I go, the more you seem to be able to control the puck." I had the ability and as long as Christy didn't go too fast, the refs couldn't discriminate against the "Special Olympic" players for having a pusher speeding around the rink.

After collecting my first seven assists that season (two during this tournament), I finally scored my first Ontario Sledge Hockey Association (OSHA) goal against the Windsor Ice Bullets at the 2006 London's Tournament. Unfortunately, we didn't make the quarter-final that year, but I learned so much playing on a higher level.

Christy's friends were in London to come to watch us play. After our game, the pretty girls and I went out for dinner, leaving my jealous teammates behind. After dinner, some of my teammates crashed at Christy's and enjoyed some drinks together. The girls let it slip that my nickname was "Muffin." There's really no origin story of the nickname other than it was pulled out of thin air one day by my team and was used to describe someone who is charming or attractive. It didn't take long for the word to get out and before I knew it, I was "Muffin" on and off the ice. I think the guys were just jealous that I had girls coming out to our games. My dad even came up with a fictitious massage therapist from Montreal named Candy LaFlossé who would meet me at my house after games for some full-body relief.

As the season ended, Christy and I kept in touch and would go out for lunch together. She's not someone who tolerated stupidity or ignorance from anybody and hated when servers would look through me when I tried to place my order, only speaking to her like I was invisible. She would tell people straight up what she thought and would tell them to open their ears and listen to what I was trying to say instead of writing me off.

Christy always reminded me that I am a force to be reckoned with. She really adored my "I'll find a way even if you don't think I can" attitude. She would tell me that I was "fierce, determined and contagiously happy."

Playing in the Big Time

The sledge hockey team I played for, the Hamilton "Bar-Ken" Sledgehammers, had an awesome opportunity in late December 2006 to play in the HSBC Arena in Buffalo, New York, home of the Buffalo Sabres. It was a pretty neat experience to play in an official NHL arena, to say the least. I can say for sure that we had a lot of ice to play on and we all felt like we were living the life of an NHL player. We beat the home team, the Buffalo Sabres (obviously named after the NHL team), 3-2 in an aggressive game that included three penalties. One of those penalties was courtesy of our goaltender Mitch, who slashed a Buffalo player across his arm for being in his crease.

For those who stayed the night in Buffalo after our game, we attended the Buffalo Sabres–Atlanta Thrashers game, where we witnessed an incredible win by the Sabres. After the game, we headed back to the hotel to hang out and have a few beers. Our captain, Chad, was laying on a bed and I was at the end of it chatting away and watching *Little People, Big World*. Since I was sitting on the bed, I couldn't hold my beer properly, so Chad's wife, Crystal, kindly held it and gave me a sip when I asked for one. A few sips after she volunteered, I looked at her with my wicked humour and said, "Hey, lady, beer me!" She looked at me like "Oh, really?" and began attacking me. Chad rolled his eyes and said, "Geez, do you guys want the room to yourself?"

Our coach Peter's twin brother, Bob, burst through the door and jokingly yelled, "What the hell is going on here, are you guys done?" After the room calmed down, he explained how we played a good game that afternoon only to finish by pointing directly at me, making me momentarily fear for my future in sledge hockey. "You! You had a perfect opportunity to score a goal. I said to myself, 'Why didn't he shoot the puck? Oh shit! That's right! He doesn't have the use of his right arm!'" Everyone in the room exploded with laughter. I actually fell off the bed onto the floor because I was laughing so hard. The setup and punchline were just too good.

The weekend was such an entertaining getaway for all of us, especially me. I was extremely thankful to experience it without my parents being there. It was one of the first times that I was able to experience what it's like to be independent with just my friends. I really needed that time away from my parents to be able to make my own choices. You don't have to explain yourself and can just be plain stupid if you want to be. Even though the hockey team is made up of people of all ages, we blended together and showed each other respect. That weekend, we played our hearts out on the ice and chilled with each other off of it.

My Sporting Career

Zeroes to Sledge Heroes

In March 2008, my team earned a championship spot. Since we had the same season record as Whitby, we had a game to see which top two teams would host the final game. My dad was pushing me for this game since my friend, Blake, was unable to attend. In the middle of the game, a Whitby player purposely ran into my dad's ankle. He went down, knocking his knee and hip out. While he was down, he looked up to see if the player was empathetic for what they had done, but the player had this guilty look on his face like it was done purposely. My dad had a hard time getting up but managed to get to the bench for a breather, and we could all see that he wasn't okay. Even my dad thought he had broken his ankle.

Coach Doug was very concerned and kept asking my dad if he was okay. Even though they say to keep your skates on to keep the swelling down, my dad undid his skate to reveal massive swelling. Coach Doug looked over to check on him again but ended up blurting out, "Holy shit!" after seeing the shape my dad's foot was in. Even though my dad was in tremendous pain, he managed to drive us home safely after we lost the game, giving Whitby the home team advantage. My dad ended up being okay mostly because of the skate. The accident caused ligament issues, swelling and bruising, and it actually took two years for the ankle to get back to a normal state. The Doctor told him that healing would have been easier if it had been broken.

Unfortunately, Whitby won the game, which meant they would host the championship game. Their home games were on Sundays and that put us at a disadvantage because we were automatically missing three players (father and sons) who didn't play due to religious obligations. We had to decide if we wanted to replace those missing players or make it up by spending more time on the ice. Thankfully we didn't have to make that decision. Our feisty manager, Shirls fought for what was fair and asked that the game be switched to a Saturday. Her tenacity paid off because the association switched the day for us to make sure we had a full team on the ice.

Our championship game against the Whitby Steelhawks in Oshawa, Ontario, was set to take place on Saturday, March 29th, 2008, at the General Motors Centre. When the day arrived, some of us met at a gas station so we could form a caravan to the arena. My teammate James (who is a brother of our assistant captain and is "able-bodied") drove with me because my friend/pusher Blake had an exam that day. We had a solid, non-stop conversation all the way there. At one point, James complimented me by saying, "There's no doubt about it, you have a great hockey IQ and you're only using one arm. You know exactly where you can help out the most and always make the right play. I truly believe that if you had your say, you would be the ultimate weapon on the ice and would absolutely be on the Canada Men's National Sledge Hockey Team." I appreciated the compliment, but it made me feel like I was once again losing out because of my lack of control in my upper torso. I know I would have made it. I would have tried my hardest and wouldn't have given up.

After a three-hour drive, we finally made it to our destination. We had plenty of time to view the ice and do some exercises before heading to our dressing room. We were all in the locker room trying to relax before the big game, but our coaches came in to hype us up.

"Let's go out there and take every effort and opportunity you have to tire the hell out of them," said Coach Doug. "Get a good lead then just relax and play our game."

Coach Peter finished by saying, "When you have the puck, they can't score!"

Moments before the puck drop, the Sledgehammers huddled around our goal crease for a quick chant.

"What time is it?" asked Chad.

"It's hammer time!" we all cheered back.

The coaches started the game with my line mates, David playing centre and AJ and I as wingmen. The three of us had been line mates since I joined the team and we built a unique connection that often led to ridiculous plays and goals. Whitby had the puck in our zone but failed to get past our defenceman with a block off his shin pads. Our defenceman, James, passed the puck to me as I cut through centre ice and navigated around the Steelhawks player with it. As I passed the blue line in their zone, knowing that David was skating parallel to me, I made a drop pass as he crossed paths behind me to throw the Hawks off. David picked up the puck and took a shot just outside the right faceoff circle. It flew in just over the Steelhawk goalie's shoulder to give us a 1-0 lead.

With less than six minutes left in the first period, our captain Chad and his line mates were on the ice keeping the puck in the Steelhawks' zone. The Steelhawks had an opportunity to get the puck out of their zone but failed as our defenceman James kept the puck in to shoot from the point. The puck bounced off the goalie and became loose as Chad took a shot in front of the net to make it a 2-0 lead.

We continued to dominate into the second period and made sure we didn't make any mistakes or let them in our zone for too long. We gained a 3-0 lead when the second period ended after David got us another goal with his "magic hands." With a good lead going into the third period and using up a lot of the Steelhawks' energy, we were confident in our game. We relaxed and played the game on our terms.

To nobody's surprise, our team tough guy, Andy (also known as Chooch), decided to take a minor penalty for roughing with a Steelhawk player near the end of the game. It was a known thing on our team that if Andy had an opposing player to mouth off to while in the penalty box, he would push it until it resulted in a fight. As I was on the bench waiting for my next shift later in the game, we saw Andy getting mixed up in a corner on the far side of the ice. Coach Doug immediately dropped his gloves and skated across the ice to prevent the situation from blowing up; however, my teammates Andrew, Steven and I saw it a little differently. As Coach Doug returned to the bench, he noticed that we were laughing hysterically and asked what our deal was. We explained that it was just the way he dropped his gloves on the spot to rush into the action. He laughed at how we saw the play-by-play and said, "With my past experience playing for the Kitchener Rangers, I was used to reacting quickly."

With less than two minutes left in the game, everyone on the bench was jumping up and down excited for the win... well, more like bobbing up and down because we were all still strapped to our sledges. We shut them out 3-0. When the air horn blew off to end the game, our team was the 2008 OSHA champions. The win was made even sweeter because the Steelhawks had mauled us at the beginning of the season with a devastating 8-3 loss. They even laughed in our faces after the game. This was payback and we only gave them two shots on net the whole game by playing the best defensive game we could muster. That season, we went from being the last-place team to the champions. That's a storybook ending.

2007–2008 Regular Season Record

W	L	P	GF	GA	TPP	PPG	PP%	TPM	PK%	HOME	AWAY
4	4	8	38	22	8	3	38%	12/18	72%	3-1	1-3

2008 London Tournament Record

W	L	P	GF	GA	TPP	PPG	PP%	TPM	PK%
-	3	3.5	1	4	10	-	-	3/5	60%

2008 Playoffs Season Record

W	L	GF	GA	TPP	PPG	PP%	TPM	PK%	HOME	AWAY
3	-	11	-	4	3	75%	3/3	100%	2-0	1-0

Quarter-Final: Peterborough Patriots — Won 3-0
Semi-Final: Mississauga Silver Streak — Won 5-0
Host the Final: Whitby Steelhawks — Lost 6-1
FINAL: Whitby Steelhawks — WON 3-0

Sledge hockey is a great sport for people who have physical disabilities or mobility challenges. Being on the ice gave all of us freedom. To us, we felt like we were playing in the NHL since we travelled and played against people from all over the world. I am so grateful to have had an amazing experience playing sledge hockey and having been part of a team of players who overcame numerous obstacles in their personal lives only to come together to give everything they had on and off the ice. We all had our ups and downs throughout the years, and even had many laughs and a few disagreements in the dressing room or on the ice. However, there were two things that kept us together as a team: respect and a sense of family.

New OSHA Season

After winning the OSHA Championship, our long-time coaches Doug and Peter along with the acting manager decided to resign from their duties; they certainly went out on a high note. With the disappointing news and short notice before the next season, our goaltender stepped in as a manager and his dad as an interim coach, along with a father of a new player on our team stepping up as assistant coach.

My friend Blake couldn't be my full-time pusher this season due to his school and work schedules. Yet again, I needed to find someone to be my legs on the ice. I started thinking about who I could ask and we happened to know this wonderful family through Stirling's soccer team that we had grown close with over the years. I had a strong connection with the father of the family, Sean, who agreed to be my pusher.

After losing four of our unique players, we gained two new players with one being Sean, who was a former rugby player. The first time Sean practised with the team, we all thought, "Thank goodness he's on our team," because we wouldn't want to be on the receiving end of what he's giving.

All these hockey stories seem to take place during the London Blizzard Tournament, but some of my best moments really did happen during those games, I swear. In the 2009 tournament, our first game was against the Peterborough Patriots. The referee for that game was standing in the hallway in front of our dressing room before the game, looked at us and said, "Oh, it's you guys, Hamilton." He obviously knew who we were because we had this same ref in the past and had a few issues with calls he made.

Of course, during the game, I exchanged words with the referees over a "Pusher Rule," one of which I mentioned in a previous story. Another rule is that pushers aren't allowed to take steps backward unless it's to get a player out of harm's way. Sean would pull me out of areas that I was jammed into to get us turned around, but that was about it. During my shift, I came around from behind the Patriots' net with the puck and got wedged between two players and the goalie, who was a few feet away. Sean had no choice but to pull me out. The whistle blew and we got two minutes for a delay of the game. Arguments ensued with my coaches defending the decision by pointing out that my stick had snapped from being hit so hard.

We had a few discussions with other referees throughout the tournament and they couldn't believe that we received a penalty for such a thing. Oh well! We did well and made it to the semi-final against the North Bay Ice Breakers over a heartbreaking 5-3 loss.

Kyle N. Scott

Stepping Up Our Sledge Hockey Game

After playing a season with the interim coaching staff that filled in for our previous coaches who had retired, our goaltender/manager, Mitch, began looking for new leadership for the following season. He found a guy named Terry who was interested in coaching the team. Previously, he had coached both a Greater Toronto Hockey League and Triple-A team.

They arranged ice time so Terry could see what we were capable of. For an hour and ten minutes, he had us doing all kinds of drills and plays. Some we've never tried before and others we've never seen before. The practice ended with twenty minutes of scrimmage to learn our individual hockey IQs. After an hour and a half of being run into the ice, we were exhausted to the point of collapsing onto the floor, which some of us did. Despite this, we were all excited about the prospect of being coached by Terry, who agreed to join our team.

My teammate Sean voiced what many of us had already concluded: Terry was serious about his coaching and wanted to build us into a winning team. From that moment on, we all knew Coach Terry wasn't going to be easy on us and was going to challenge us to be the best sledge hockey players we could be. Once we got to know Terry, we found that as tough as he was on the ice, he was just as much a softie off it. Coach Terry was a man with a heart of gold and knew how to draw the potential out of his players.

With Terry leading the way, we entered a new season in the fall. My friend Sean was no longer able to push me after moving to Acton, Ontario, due to his demanding work schedule. Even though I knew how much he loved sledge hockey and hated having to quit, I understood where he was coming from. After our last practice together, Sean, my dad and I walked toward the parking lot to notice that it was raining heavily. My dad went to pull the van around while I waited with Sean. As I was getting in, my front wheels got caught on the lifted ramp and I went sailing off of it onto the wet ground. A lady who saw the whole incident pulled up behind us, got out of her car and said, "Who are these people? They should be fired for being so careless!" Sean felt terrible about it, you could see it on his face. My dad explained what had happened and who they were. While I was still on the ground laughing at the situation. If anything, the lady just delayed the time it took for me to get up off the ground.

I was on the hunt yet again for a new pusher. In college, I switched courses and had a whole new pool of students to ask. There was this young whippersnapper (by whippersnapper, I mean full of energy, goes after what he wants and a loud Frenchman) by the name of Steven who was in my History of Architecture class. He always said hello to me and went out of his way to introduce himself one day. He agreed to play sledge hockey with me after I sent him an email sometime later detailing what was involved and the schedule. The first practice we had really impressed him. He was amazed by what I could do playing with only one hand, and how accurate and aggressive I was with the puck. Two weeks later, my mom picked up Steven for a tournament in Brampton.

After a month and a half playing under Coach Terry, we quickly learned a whole new meaning for the word "teamwork." We had communication, respect and work ethic drilled into us. His goal was clear: to teach hockey in a systematic manner that he thought would benefit every player. Confidence would be gained by the acquisition of knowledge and he wanted to teach us how to perform like any highly developed team. He saw us make great strides and improvements weekly.

During our first home game of the season against Toronto, Coach Terry put me out for a penalty kill. We managed to keep the puck out of our zone. My teammate Sean passed me the puck from our end as I made my way toward Toronto's net. One of the defencemen was forechecking me in an attempt to make me lose control of the puck. I managed to bodycheck him in response with my right shoulder to stave him off and shoot the puck in, a shorthanded goal and our first goal of the period.

Later in the game, I came off the bench and hollered for a pass from one of my teammates, Delly. Delly saw me wide open at centre ice and flipped me the puck through the air. I snagged the puck and took off on a breakaway, managing to trick the goalie by sending the puck to the roof of the net. I thought that was an amazing play started by a get-go pass from Delly. We ended up slaughtering Toronto with a 9-2 win.

Kyle N. Scott

Biggest Hit on Ice

There was changes surrounding the 2010 season of sledge hockey. The Hamilton intermediate team I joined a few years back was folding due to a lack of player interest and a Brantford team that was soaking up most of our players. They weren't poaching anybody; it was just part of the rules. You had to join the team that was closest to you and approximately 90 percent of the Hamilton team was from Brantford. It was even uncertain whether Coach Terry was able to return. No players meant no team.

The president of our association set up a meeting for both of Hamilton's intermediate teams to discuss how they were going to combine into one. Some of my teammates who live in Hamilton were unhappy about this change and couldn't join the team. I became a new player on the Hamilton Score Sledgehammers (named after the sports network The Score). I also took on a new pusher, Andrew, who I had gone to high school with after Steven could no longer commit.

That December, we were playing against the Kitchener K-W Sidewinders in a very physical game. I was in front of the Sidewinders' net, trying to distract the goalie to tip in the puck or at least wait for my teammates to pass for a shot. The goalie and I were exchanging words with each other because he didn't like the fact that I had a pusher. People still don't seem to understand that having a pusher is set in stone. Any athlete who can't otherwise move a sledge is allowed to have a pusher. The pusher becomes a player on the ice who is able to play in the neutral and attacking zones without ice limitations.

However, pushers are not allowed to play within an area in their defensive zone bounded by the area with lines drawn from the defending goalposts to faceoff spots and out to intersect with the blue line. Confusing, I know, but we knew the rules. Despite this, the opposing goalie kept telling us to follow the rules, but we stayed anyway to piss him off, knowing we were within our rights to do so.

Anyway, hanging around the net paid off because my teammate shot the puck from the blue line. The puck bounced off the goalie and I chased it, took a shot and scored as the goalie dived for it. He went bonkers and tried to start a fight with me. That didn't work, so he went to the refs to complain

My Sporting Career

about the pusher rules. Then tensions boiled over and the coaches from both teams started going at it. In the madness, the ref called the goal off because he didn't know the pusher rules. Now I was pissed off because the ref didn't know how to do his job. We managed to edge out Kitchener 3-2 and I got an assist on one of them.

Even though I wasn't playing on the team I wanted to play on, I still gave it my all. I still had a passion for the game, but my connection to the team wasn't. When the London Blizzard Tournament came up again, we went in with a poor record after playing lousy. But that changed during the tournament. We added more players from Brantford who wanted to play and a former teammate, Sean, made his way back. I was happy for his arrival because not only was he a great guy, his aggressive nature and competitiveness were sorely needed on the ice.

The first game was against the Sarnia Ice Hawks, whom we dominated 7-1. The second game was very close at 1-0 for us against the Northumberland Predators. The third game was a very intense and aggressive game against the Peterborough Patriots where I scored an unseen game-winning goal to take a 4-3 win.

After winning all three games, we clinched first place and advanced straight to the semi-final game against the Sudbury Northern Sliders. The game was a nail-biter that went beyond overtime into a shootout. The pressure was on with all of us knowing what was at stake: possible championship gold. We won 2-1 in the shootout, with our goaltender saving all three shots for our team, and advanced to the finals.

Even though I have championship experience when we won it in 2008 with my former team, I hadn't had the opportunity to make it to the finals in any of the tournaments. The championship game was against the North Bay Ice Breakers, who have always been a strong team.

The Ice Breakers came out very strong in the first period with a soul-crushing 4-0 lead. The game became more aggressive and physical during the second period, which saw the biggest clean hit I ever made on someone who was twice the size of me. We collided head-to-head along the boards with our sticks flying into the air. It took him several seconds to get back up before he skated back to the bench, all the while mouthing off to me. That same guy was mouthing off to me during the first period so he deserved every bit of pain that came with that hit. My pusher Andrew gave me water once we were back on the bench and I asked if that guy was still fuming. Andrew confirmed he was, which made me happy because it was a solid check.

The Ice Breakers scored two more goals in the second and added two more in the third. We were annihilated 8-0, but we got second place, which is something to be proud of. We were happy with the effort we put out and had a great run in that tournament.

Cruisers Cup Tournament

A few days after my nonna's burial, there was a sledge hockey tournament. I was down and didn't want to play, but I knew my nonna would want me to play and enjoy myself. It was the first weekend of November 2011 and the Cruisers Cup Tournament was being held in Brampton, Ontario. One of my teammates, Cam, put tape on the back of my helmet that read "Nonna" and told me to play for her.

The first game was against our biggest rival, the Mississauga Silver Streaks. We knew going into it that it would be a very emotional and physical game with all the blood that had been spilled over the years. After two periods, the Silver Streaks had a 3-2 lead. Halfway through the third, we were still losing by a goal and had lots of chances, but the puck just didn't want to go in. At two minutes left in the third, we pulled our goalie to get an extra attacker to try to at least tie up the game. The coaches put me on as the extra attacker since I was known for setting up plays and goals. We managed to keep the puck in their zone for a while and kept it under our protection while everyone got in position. My pusher, Andrew, positioned me behind the net and, as we made our way around, the goalie slid over to the other side of the net. We had tricked him into thinking I was going to do a wrap-around goal. We skated a few feet ahead and passed the puck under my sledge so the defencemen couldn't see it. The goalie must have thought I was going to score by going behind the net with the puck I didn't have because my teammate, Billy, was perfectly positioned on the opposite side to shoot the puck in. That goal forced the game into overtime, which ran out the clock for a tie game anyway.

The second game was against the Buffalo Sabres. After the first period, we took a 2-0 lead. However, the next two periods got more aggressive and we made several mistakes that cost us a 5-2 loss. The third game was against the Ottawa Valley Bandits, who were a very strong and skilled team. Despite their talent, we managed to shut them out in all three periods and beat them 4-0. After playing three games with a win, loss and tie, we had enough points to make it to the quarter-final against our other rivals, the Mississauga Red Dawgs. (I'm not sure if both rivalries being with Mississauga is a coincidence or if it's something in their water.) They took an early lead in the first period, but we just couldn't get it going and fell behind each period with a 5-1 loss. We took home second place yet again, but at least it's a podium finish.

Ending My Sledge Hockey Career... Unexpectedly

Sadly, in October 2012, I was forced to retire from sledge hockey because of my hip dysplasia. I admit that this was really heartbreaking to have no choice but to walk away from a game I loved so much. It honestly took me a few years to overcome the frustration and depression of not being able to play. I really was crushed and still miss being able to play today.

I have been lucky enough to play in 138 games over the fifteen years of my sledge hockey career. However, I sometimes reminisce about the last game I ever played on November 20th, 2011. We were playing Niagara and were down four goals within the first five minutes of the game. Things got dicey with fights breaking out. Half of my team was ejected before the end of the period, leaving only seven players left to play. I ended up having thirty minutes of ice time and played with an injured hand. It wasn't my ideal game to end my career on, but I didn't have a choice. I had plenty of ice time, though, and that made the game memorable.

Even though I knew my career was coming to an end sooner rather than later, I wish I was more prepared for it. It still hurts to think about and I think it always will. Having said all that, I'm extremely grateful and thankful for the opportunity to play on a hockey team for so long and to play against people from all over North America and overseas. I truly enjoyed every moment of it, on and off the ice.

CAREER STATS WITH HAMILTON J.R. SLEDGEHAMMERS 1996-2005

GP	G	A	P	P.I.M.
50	18	33	51	24

SEASON CAREER STATS WITH HAMILTON BAR-KEN SLEDGEHAMMERS 2005-2010

GP	G	A	P	P.I.M.
64	11	42	53	16

PLAYOFF CAREER STATS

GP	G	A	P	P.I.M.
9	1	5	6	2

SEASON CAREER STATS WITH HAMILTON SCORE SLEDGEHAMMERS 2010-2011

GP	G	A	P	P.I.M.
14	6	8	14	4

PLAYOFF CAREER STATS

GP	G	A	P	P.I.M.
1	-	-	-	-

SEASON CAREER STATISTICS

GP	G	A	P	P.I.M.
78	17	50	67	20

PLAYOFF CAREER STATISTICS

GP	G	A	P	P.I.M.
10	-	5	5	2

Chapter 6: Living with CP — Emotionally

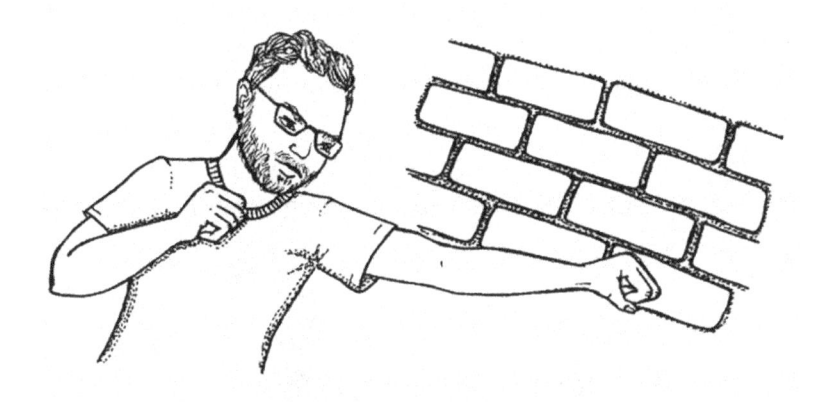

First Emotional Breakdown

Throughout my life, I have experienced many emotional breakdowns. The first one I can recall was on a Saturday night at the beginning of 2005, at the age of fifteen.

Everything came to a boiling point and I felt overwhelmed and frustrated. I was sitting at the bottom of my basement stairs, terribly upset, asking question after question to my dad. Why was my type of CP such a mystery? Why did I even fight to stay alive? Why am I even here? Would it have been better if I hadn't made it? I was feeling left out of all these things I saw people doing like partying, having girlfriends and getting jobs. All those teenage milestones kids my age were supposed to be hitting weren't happening for me.

Some of you reading this might think I'm being too hard on myself and that's okay, but know that it wasn't from a lack of trying to get out there. I had asked girls out and the answer was always "no" or they were already taken. It wasn't because of my personality. I often spoke to my best friend James and a few others about it, and knowing full well the issue was not as simple as being viewed as a friend. It was my disability. My disability was once again preventing me from experiencing something I felt was important to me. It was like a punch in the face as everything started to come to a head.

I would sit there and just replay everything I should have been able to do and experience over and over in my head. I needed to find myself, my potential and to learn to love me for me. I didn't want to let CP define me as a person. My dad gave me the best advice, "You don't have arms, you don't have legs, but you've been given the most valuable gift of all, your brain. If you have that, you have it all. You can be strategic and plan your future. Know how to go after your dreams and make them come true."

Transitioning into Adulthood with My Disability

As I transitioned into adulthood, my daily frustrations would occasionally develop into a full meltdown, leaving me emotionally drained.

There are said to be four stages to the human life cycle. I believe as a twenty-year-old, I'm in the second stage, which is self-discovery, enterprise and adventurousness. It basically covers adolescence, early adulthood and adulthood. I've completed post-secondary education, volunteered, travelled and discovered new things, but my options have been limited. Most of my generation were starting their lives in many ways.

Those years were challenging for me because in my mind I knew I could do a lot more. I'm a determined person and I won't allow anyone, including myself, to stop me. If my options weren't limited, I would have done some travelling around the world during my early twenties with one of my friends or cousins. The same with dating. I know if I wasn't in this situation I would have been in a monogamous relationship. I'm not saying this because I deserve it or anything, but because of my charming personality. Some of you may think that no one could ever know the outcomes if things were different. That might be true, but I can assure you that many more opportunities would have been available to me like they are for able-bodied people. Those opportunities just aren't there for those with tougher disabilities.

At this point in life, I should have been experiencing different milestones like dancing to a love song at a wedding or function with my partner, going on a date night or going away with friends and so forth. I'm happy that I'm seeing these things in general; however, I only hope that I will get to experience it myself one day.

I'm extremely thankful to be living in a technological world to stay connected with everyone who is a part of my life.

Losing Patience

In my mid-twenties, I went through a series of meltdowns. I knew I had a major support system built around family, friends and community members, but there's only so much people can do. I have pushed myself in sports and education, and in search of independence. I dig way down inside to find something to be proud of, so I can appreciate what I do have and push forward for a better tomorrow. But every day of my life, I deal with the demands of living a "normal life."

Most people have no idea what goes through my mind on a daily basis. There are days and weeks where sleeping is a major chore. My mind plays tricks on me. I know my mind is normal, but I have desires and needs like everyone else. However, expressing them is not always an option. You can get the assistance needed to complete most tasks, albeit simple ones, such as having a snack. I either have to ask someone to do it for me or just wait. Most times that snack never materializes because I lose patience and interest, with my wait outliving my desire for food.

Stop and think of how many tasks you perform independently in a 24-hour window. Can you imagine having to wait for at least 98 percent of them to be fulfilled? What about going out with your friends or close cousins without your parents being there to help? Having your parents taking you to your date with a girl you've never met before? Think about it. I always have to depend on others to get me to locations and pick me up. Where is my privacy? Things can easily be taken for granted when you're able-bodied.

Most people have their day planned out for themselves: family, personal commitments, socializing... and in all that, they have to fit me in somewhere to connect with me. Most of the time, my days are structured around social events that I have no choice but to be a part of. I am not saying that I don't enjoy the social surroundings. I would like to make my own choices in life like how I spend my time being entertained or what I do with my friends or with sports or dating.

I deal with this situation a minute at a time. I'm frustrated, concerned for the future, yearning for independence, looking toward future goals and the happiness of having my own family. That is why I know I'm normal in my thinking; I just want what most people want. I'm getting tired of always fighting to stay positive, keeping my dreams alive, being happy, always putting that smile on for people who praise me. It stings when I'm always told to be patient, I'm not the only one out there, things will come to those who wait.

It wasn't about dealing with cerebral palsy. It was about the walls and barriers I needed to knock down in order for me to move forward in pursuing what I deserved. Some may think I am envious or jealous, and it does feel that way at times, but I'm not. These are all emotions we express and experience in life. We just learn to control them in time. It would be nice to be independent, so I could just once find out what it would be like to do whatever I wanted to do, even if only for a day. I think everyone with a disability wishes for something like that. What blind person wouldn't want to see for a day just to experience what the majority of the world does?

Emotionally, my overall frustration is that I feel behind in my life: getting a job, moving out on my own, home ownership, relationships, marriage, kids, life... the list continues. I understand when people say, "The right girl will come along," or "That one didn't deserve you," but how long can I keep hearing that phrase and when will it happen? You can only hold hope for so long.

I know in my heart and soul that I would have accomplished everything I desperately feel like I should have by now if everyone could see past my cerebral palsy. It's the first and last thing a lot of people see, and that creates a lot of assumptions that, ultimately, closes many doors for me.

Struggling with Questions

In my late twenties, I had a lot of thoughts of intimacy going around in my mind (not that I haven't thought about it years prior). I know I'm not the only one, but I feel like my situation is a lot more complicated than most.

I kept asking if I would ever have my own life. To have the feeling of meeting a special woman who would love me for who I am. Would I ever get the feeling of intimacy, holding hands while sitting at a table or putting my hand on her legs when at a restaurant? Having sex whenever we decided to and not even having to consider paying for it?

Will I work like everyone else? Having that feeling of being independent and having an income. Having a place of my own whether it's as a homeowner or renting. Having a wedding that I've always dreamed of and being surrounded by everyone in my life to see me wed the love of my life. Being able to experience what it's like to be a father and having a family of my own.

Opportunities to experience and explore with my friends and cousins without having my parents watch over me all the time. Will I ever get an opportunity to say that I'm seeing someone/have a girlfriend or got a job?

Over the years, I've had to live vicariously through some of my friends' and cousins' lives to experience what it's like to be a part of these types of things. However, having said that, I'm grateful for the things that I've been able to do. I just wish I had a chance to do more things for myself. Will that day ever come?

Kyle N. Scott

Reflecting on the "What If?"

Over the years, many people I meet have asked me, "How do you cope with CP?" and "How does it affect your life?" Well, it affects every part of my life and I find things that help take my mind off it. For example, most kids from my generation played video games because they were fun, but for me, it had a different meaning. Not only was it a way to cope, but it was also a way to regain some control. I manipulated my character to do what I wanted them to do as if I were in the game. It was freeing. I love sports, so I mostly played sports games, especially after my hip became an issue. Just playing games for a few hours a week provided an escape.

For me, coping with CP isn't the issue because I'm still able to be involved in many activities with family and friends. When I run into an obstacle, I always find another way. The hardest part to cope with is actually how much CP has affected my goals and dreams in life, and they've been affected in so many different ways. Even though I've overcome a lot in my life, I can't help but ask, "What if?"

There are days and nights when I often think of where I would be in life if I were not in this situation. Where would I have gone for my post-secondary education, university or college? Which city would have I done my studying in? Would I have gone out of the city? Would I still be an architectural technician or in another profession? Would I have become a homeowner by myself or with someone else? Who would I have dated? Would I have been married and had a family before I reached thirty? These are the questions I've struggled with over the years.

I will admit that CP or even the type of CP that I have (athetoid) has taken away milestones that I would have liked to have reached throughout my life. Things most people experience like getting a job as a teenager or working as a hockey referee. During post-secondary, would I have become a waiter or bartender at a place like The Keg? I heard they pay well and give students a lot of flexibility with their studies.

You might be asking why I would bother asking these "What if?" questions. Why would I put myself down? Maybe you think I should be more grateful and proud of my accomplishments — *which I am*. I don't see it that way. I'm not putting myself down or setting myself up for failure by thinking about these things. I feel like I'm being realistic — and who doesn't dream of what could have been?

I've always been more mature than my age. I've always been determined and I knew exactly what I wanted out of life at a very young age. With my personal motivation and drive, I am sure I would have been successful in accomplishing the goals I set for myself. Just look at what I've accomplished in terms of overcoming the obstacles that I've had to face. If those obstacles weren't there, all my energy could have been focused on doing something more constructive or creative. Neither you nor I will ever know the answers to the "What if?" questions. I just have to work with what I have.

While this time is full of reflections, the most important thing is that I'm grateful for meeting some amazing people: instructors, educational assistants and colleagues like Steven, who has become a lifetime friend.

The Reality of Being a Child with CP

Starting from day one of development, I was just a baby who needed normal baby attention. Feedings on demand, diaper changes and normal bonding through visual, auditory and physical contact. Doctors followed my development for the first year of my life. Being born into the stressful situation that I was in, it was a requirement to have quarterly visits with doctors so they could keep track of my mental and physical development, cognitive abilities and motor skills.

My parent's world changed around the eighteen-month mark. Through multiple meetings with several specialists, I was eventually diagnosed with cerebral palsy. This is when the floodgates opened for therapists — OTs, physiotherapists, speech therapists, you name it — to start working with me. My parents went into fight mode, getting all the professional advice and best medical care possible. This was both challenging for me as a patient and for them as parents. Their perseverance was all so I could be my best physically, mentally and socially. The programs I was in allowed me to think outside the box, to think creatively, and know that one day I could reach for my goals. It was just one day at a time.

Everyone who helped me along the way — therapists, teacher's assistants, friends and family — supported and challenged me every day. Those who know me know I'm a force to be reckoned with and my determination is unstoppable. Everyone in my support system had no choice but to learn along the way like I did. But I showed them that we could get there and that there were no boundaries.

I leaned heavily on my village of support. We had to tap into the resources available to us and we really had to dig and unearth these opportunities because they certainly don't come to you. You quickly learn what's available, and more times than not, what's not available. Networking and being socially active with everyone you come into contact with was really a key component because you never know what others know. Maybe they've gone through something similar or similar enough that you could benefit from it too. Maybe they know someone who has experienced the same things you have. Maybe someone comes up with a brilliant idea you never thought of that opens the door to something amazing.

My parents used resources provided by the Children's Developmental Rehabilitation Program at the Chedoke Hospital in Hamilton, Ontario. The program offered a parent support group to those caring for special needs children. It was a ten-week course called the Hannon Group, which facilitated a speech reinforcement program that helped parents strategize ways to develop their child's speech patterns.

After the first five sessions, parents had to self-reflect by watching themselves interact with their children on video. This gave them an opportunity to see where they could improve what they were taught in the classes. The therapists would also provide feedback to make sure everyone was doing their best to help their child's development, while also giving positive reinforcement to ensure parents knew that what they were doing was of great benefit.

The group itself was made up of various disabilities, from mild to moderate. The parents had an opportunity to bond in class and continued to meet a once a month, which was basically a night out for everyone. It was like a support group where everyone could vent and talk about what they were going through with people who actually understood their situation.

Living with CP — Emotionally

Battling through all the emotions, rough patches and challenging moments through the years gave me resolve. I always knew that tomorrow would be a new day. I would meet new people, have new opportunities, maybe be lucky enough to come across a new advancement in medicine that could help me gain some independence. I've routinely reached out to those I could confide in when I was going through a turbulent time. I knew that I would need my family and close friends to help deal with my concerns and thoughts. Using social media is another great outlet. Being able to stay in touch with family and friends virtually has been helpful.

My advice to anyone going through hard times, no matter what it is, is to talk it out. Don't hold it in. Don't dwell on the negativity and push yourself to the brink silently. Reach out to family and friends you know you can trust and those who will be truthful and respectful with you. Together, you can work through whatever you're going through to find answers. You can seek professional help or maybe go to church for some religious counselling. Connect with your support village and stay in contact with as many people as you can. Socialize with those who will inspire you to be the best you can be. They will lift you up and help bolster a more positive outlook toward life.

People see me in a wheelchair and probably think of the challenges I have to endure, but that's something I'm already painfully aware of every day when I look at other people and wonder what challenges they must face. As much as I want people to look past my disability, I hope it gets people to pause so they can appreciate what they have. There's a quote by author Wendy Mass that says, "Be kind, for everyone you meet is fighting a battle you know nothing about." Acknowledging those seen and unseen struggles in others helps shift the focus of my own struggles and inspires me to keep fighting, keep living, remain positive and hopefully inspire others. So, put on those leather boxing gloves and get in the ring called life. When the bell rings, fight the good fight and come out a champion!

Chapter 7: Living with CP — Physically

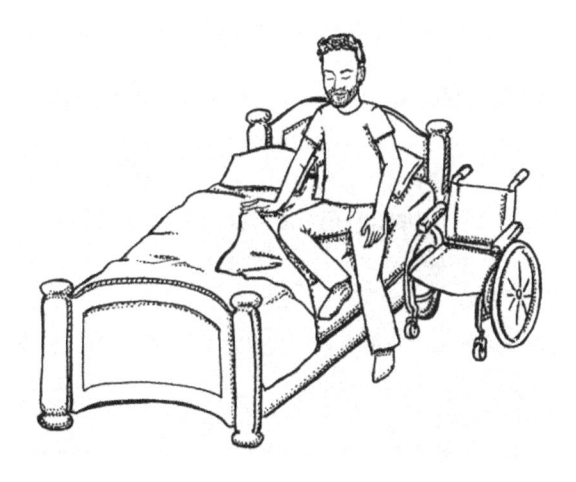

Involuntary Movements

During one of our yearly trips to Florida, I began noticing changes in my body. This wasn't a puberty thing, but rather focused on my CP. We were at a restaurant with our cousin George Junior and a few of his friends eating and listening to a live band. I've never had full control over my body, but I could feel myself making involuntary and jerky movements while sitting in my chair. I told my dad that something was going on with me that I had never experienced before.

We found out later that because of my spastic CP, my body would move involuntarily based on my emotions. So, it didn't matter if I was happy, excited, sad, angry or nervous, if the emotion was high enough, I would constantly move around. It's similar to someone who has Parkinson disease.

At first, it was really humiliating because I couldn't control myself. I began to try different strategies to see which worked best for me, like holding my hands close to my chest, putting my right hand behind or even under my butt and crossing my right leg with my left hand underneath. It took a bit of time for it to work and find control over that dang spasticity. It wasn't until my mid-twenties when I noticed that my spasticity had decreased. Each situation has been different along the way, but these strategies that I've come up with give me comfort and confidence over the movements.

So, I want you to think about this one. Have you ever been in a car holding a drink that is filled to the brim? Take off the lid while in the passenger seat and tell the driver to take you on a wild ride. Go fifty kilometres per hour down the bumpiest road you can find. By this point, you're trying not to spill the drink and all I can say is good luck with that.

Your drink will be clapping up the sides of the cup like waves crashing into a mountainside. The drink will be slapping your lips as you try to take a sip or two without spilling it on yourself. Want to make it harder? Pretend to be a bobblehead and shake your head around during the ride. Rotate your shoulders in circular motions like you're stretching. Shake your cup hand a little bit more too. It sounds funny, but that's what it's like for me whenever I want to drink out of a cup. It's a disaster. I can't stop my spasticity long enough to take a drink of water. No amount of focus can get me there. I can't even drink when someone else holds the glass; I need a straw just to have my thirst quenched.

Pain Like I've Never Felt Before

A week out from Christmas in 2011, I was getting ready to go to hockey practice. As I stepped outside of our house, my right hip completely gave out on me and I was in severe pain to the point of tears. I was on the ground yelling that I couldn't move and to get Stirling for help. He carried me to my bedroom where I spent the evening in incredible pain. I knew what happened wasn't good because the pain was more excruciating than anything I've ever experienced.

I was still in severe pain the next morning but managed to make it to the washroom. When I tried to get back into my wheelchair, I fell to the floor and passed out because of the pain. My mom had to call our friend for help because she couldn't safely lift me on her own when I was dead weight. I spent the next three days straight in bed. After that, I was stuck in a wheelchair all day every day. Since it was around Christmas, getting an appointment wasn't easy, so I was in agony on painkillers for several weeks until I finally saw someone in January.

The x-rays showed my hip was shattered looking, and the head of the femur was out of its socket. This situation makes my hip sit back further back and completely disconnected from where the bone should rest in the hip socket. I had no relief for months. I stopped the physio I was going to before the incident because I simply couldn't move around without pain. In time, my hip healed and worked itself out by finding a place to rest.

Sleeping Is Often a Nightmare

Have you ever heard people say that they love to sleep and can't wait until they head to bed at night? Well I, on the other hand, don't look forward to it at all. I sleep because I'm human and have to; otherwise I'll look like a zombie from *The Walking Dead* except I'd be wheeling around in a wheelchair. "Brainsssss. Errrrrr." Squeak, squeak!

Most nights, I don't sleep well and I'm not always well rested by morning. I'm a light sleeper, which I've unfortunately inherited from my dad. However, when I do get down to sleep, it's no more than three to four hours of tossing and turning every now and then, which prevents me from getting solid REM sleep. I start off on my stomach on top of my right hand and arm to help control my spasticity since that side is difficult to get control of. Some nights, depending on what mood I'm in or if my anxiety is up. Hyperventilating isn't exactly conducive to sleep.

I also find myself frustrated when trying to figure out how I can get ahead in life. Some nights when my anxiety is extremely high, I will take a Gravol or have a shot of my favourite Irish cream liqueur, Baileys and a glass or two... maybe three... of red wine (when I was in my mid-twenties) to take that edge off. The wheel in your mind is turning at 100 miles per hour when you're trying to relax and you need something to overpower it. However, when I'm asleep my dad has told me that I don't look like I have CP. It's almost like my body relaxes to the point of letting my muscles go back to where they should be. He says I look beyond relaxed and at peace.

Waking up in the morning isn't always pleasant. I often have a stiff neck or a kink in my shoulder blade and it varies depending on how I slept or what happened the day before. When it's severely painful, I can't function at all. It makes me feel more disabled than I already am and that's when the emotions kick in. It's terrible dealing with that pain on top of CP for twenty-four hours or more. Sometimes medication and muscle relaxants help a little bit, but it's not a sure thing.

The only good thing about sleep is being able to dream. In my early teens, I started having dreams that I was able to fully control my body and do various activities that I couldn't normally do in waking life. I could do anything you could imagine. This was way before the James Cameron movie called *Avatar* came out, but that's how I dreamt it. After I saw that movie, I couldn't believe that someone created a movie about a lot of things I had been dreaming about; it was very surreal. To be able to fly, soar above the clouds, climb up mountains, run without boundaries... what a thing to dream about. It's too bad I didn't turn my dreams into a book or movie script like James Cameron did because you might have seen me on my yacht today!

Freedom in the Water

In July 2014, we revisited Florida after a break of eight years to visit my great-aunt Jean after the loss of her husband, my great-uncle George. During that time, I had changed physically, now having hip dysplasia, which led to me losing my ability to walk and a lot of my independence.

Being in the water has always given me complete freedom and safety to move around without worrying about a fall, so I've had a lot of time in water throughout my life. There was one morning in Florida where my dad was taking me to the pool at the condo. "So, this is what my life is like now?" I said to my dad. I was thinking about it and just blurted it out, so my dad was caught off guard by such a serious question out of the blue. After he understood that my life had changed since our last visit, I remember him saying, "Yeah, this is it. Now, what are we going to do with it?" What he meant was we either moved forward or let this rule my life, ultimately leading to defeat. He assured me that I wasn't wired for defeat and that I wouldn't have made it as far as I have otherwise. Just look at all the things I've accomplished despite my challenges.

"Push through. Use your gift," he said pointing to my head. "Forget about what we can't do. We'll focus on what we can."

At that moment, I knew the only thing to do was move forward. I began swimming laps in the pool with my dad, who supported me by holding onto the back of my swimsuit. This helped me keep my mind on using my muscles to propel myself. It wasn't easy because my limbs don't naturally want to straighten out. Up and down the pool I went until I was swimming independently by that evening. I could make it to the ends of the pool like never before. "God takes one thing and gives you another," I recall my dad saying after I swam on my own.

I am at peace with having CP even if it's coined as being a "mystery one." Sure, it's taken away opportunities and has made me work harder for the simpler things, but I've overcome those challenges in the end. Hip dysplasia is the thing that has really taken away the most opportunities for me. The CP I can handle, but I feel like the dysplasia is unfair. The sheer pain is enough to drive anyone mad, but to have it prevent me from experiencing so many things in life has been too much at times. Hip dysplasia and CP are an awful combination.

I wonder if a hip operation were available to me, would I have my independence back or, at least, be more independent? If I didn't even have hip dysplasia, would I still have independence at this point in my life? What opportunities would I have had without it? Where would I be now?

Experiencing that level of freedom was exhilarating and the feeling of accomplishment made me so proud. I could now swim independently, with supervision, for exercise, socialization, independence and to get refreshed. I might not swim like everyone else, but I'm swimming nonetheless because I didn't give up.

Kyle N. Scott

Fractured

In February 2015, my power wheelchair was really starting to get old; I've had that thing since grade nine. We ordered a new one and we arranged for a DARTS bus to help us pick it up the day it came in. Since I was taking a manual chair on the bus and we were picking up a new one, my mom asked if it would be an issue to bring two chairs on. They didn't have an issue with it and off we went.

I took my new chair for a spin before the bus picked us up. When we were going to board, the driver was overly concerned about the two wheelchairs, telling us they couldn't take us home. Apparently, it was against the law to drive with an empty chair onboard. My mom explained that she called ahead to see if it was okay. The driver called their office after to see what could be done. While he was waiting for someone to give him an answer, he decided to put someone else in first and parked him right behind the driver's seat. When the driver was given the green light for the two wheelchairs, I drove mine up the bus ramp only to see that the other rider took up a ton of space. There isn't much space on the bus at the best of times because there are poles and other accessible things in the way. Between the guy and the poles, I was going to have difficulty manoeuvring. As I got to the top of the ramp and turned, I realized that my right foot was caught underneath the guy's footrest a little too late. I yelled that I was stuck and in severe pain.

The driver was trying to get me unstuck, while my mom was trying to see what was causing the pain. It was so intense that I passed out. The driver called an ambulance even though we were basically in front of a hospital. I started coming around when the paramedics arrived. They examined my foot and said I just sprained it. I knew it wasn't sprained; it was broken. They asked if I wanted to go to the hospital, but I wanted to go home and sleep even though I don't normally sleep during the day.

When I woke up, I was in unbelievable pain. When my dad came home from work that evening, he noticed that my foot was very swollen and I noticed that it was far worse than it had been hours earlier. Into the car and off to urgent care we went. Once I had x-rays done, it was confirmed that my ankle was fractured and it was suggested to get a cast. My dad was like, "No way!" and asked the doctor if she knew what it would be like to put a cast on someone who has spasticity from cerebral palsy. The doctor took my dad's advice (which was unheard of) and decided to put me in an air cast boot until I saw a surgeon. I hated all six weeks of having to wear that boot because it was super uncomfortable. Any time you have to wear something foreign on your body, it takes time to get used to before you don't notice it all; however, it was still painful to stand on whenever I needed to use the bathroom. The really funny thing about the boot was this might have been the only time where I didn't feel disabled. Most people who saw my cast thought I was in a wheelchair because of that and not CP.

Knock Me Out Botox…

To those who do not know, I have been receiving Botox injections since I was seven years old. Yes, I said, "Botox." However, it's not for aesthetic purposes, but to relax my muscles and spasticity. Both my hamstrings and abductors are injected with Botox every three months… total of six injections, three on each side.

One of the most common symptoms of cerebral palsy is muscle stiffness and spastic movements. A cerebral palsy child often struggles with spastic movements that are unpredictable and can even cause pain. There are many different treatment options, but no cure for the muscle difficulties of cerebral palsy. Botulinum toxin A, often referred to as Botox, presents a temporary treatment option via injectable therapy to reduce muscle spasticity. A toxin secreted by bacteria has been altered to be successfully and safely used in people with specific medical conditions, including cerebral palsy. It can provide significant relief for a child with limiting spastic movements, discomfort, and pain.

The Botox doctor who I went to at the time was tall and handsome with long curly hair and was in his thirties, who once told me that he decided to become a doctor rather than an architect. He mentioned that he found the course hard. I looked at him and said, "You're a doctor! and that is not hard?"

Over the years, the Botox doctor and I discovered that we wear fancy and humorous clothes. He was known for wearing fancy socks and I'm known for wearing humorous underwear... still am to this day! Even the nurse who assists the doctor looked forward to seeing what I have on that day!

One of my fondest memories of this doctor was when we decided to try the Botox on my left hand. Well, it was an interesting episode. First of all, we were in a tiny room in the basement at Chedoke Hospital without windows. Secondly, it was extremely hot in the room. Thirdly, the doctor and my mom were trying to keep my left hand still so they could find the right area to inject Botox. Well, I guess because everything happened at once and I was overheated, I passed out — out cold. However, I was aware of what was going on and heard them calling my name. Finally, after half a minute, I regained consciousness and the doctor asked how I was doing. With a big smile on my face, I started laughing. After five seconds, my mom muttered "I think I'm going to pass out now." The doctor said, "Oh no, I'm not good with people passing out," and called the nurse for assistance. They laid my mother on the bed and she came around much faster than I did. The doctor reiterated that he is not great with people passing out. We looked at him and said, "You're a doctor!"

My Botox doctor, who has been injecting me for nearly a decade, had resigned from the practice to focus on his other practice, sports medicine. It never occurred to me that I would be his last Botox patient. Lucky him or lucky me! A few seconds after I received my injection, he told me he was going to tattoo me on his arm — I've always wondered if he ever did!

Choices... Whose Choices??? Not Always a Choice

Have you ever had the unfortunate experience of being fed by someone? There is a big difference if you are given the odd grape in your mouth or a shared dessert of the same fork. There comes a point that the person who needs assistance in eating has to learn patience. You will have to wait until they are ready to feed you, whether you're hungry or not. The person feeding you has to be aware of how much to put on a fork, what the temperature of the food is to prevent burning your mouth, and how to wait for chewing, swallowing and digesting the food. The texture of the food is also important when being assisted in feeding. Take soup, for instance: as a hot liquid, it takes much more attention to make sure the person you're feeding is not wearing more of the soup than they're ingesting. The only hope is at most times you get the same person helping with the eating or trained help. I have become tolerant at most times, and have been grateful when someone is comfortable in helping me eat.

In our household, I am given choices at most times. We have a wide variety of menus, and again I am very happy with our selections. I do ask the infamous question, "What's for dinner?" That is just so I can prepare my taste buds and see whether I'm in or not on the excitement for that night's selection of food. I do throw suggestions for dinner or even lunches out there at times — just a simple request, and voilà, that's what we eat for dinner.

Obviously, my other challenges are toileting, bathing and changing. Even though it's humiliating that I need assistance, I would rather have help than spending ten minutes, or more depending on if my muscles are cooperating, and wearing jogging pants to do number uno business. Changing is probably the easiest thing to do except for the buttons. For bathing, I definitely need someone to help because it's not safe going in and out of the tub or shower. In fact, I think we all experience this factor at some point in our lives.

Even though I am given choices, I am unable to be spontaneous as to when I want and how I want my independence when it comes to a shower or a bath. Sometimes you just feel like taking a shower, but I have to make sure I have assistance. It may not be the perfect time for the person to assist me. They may be tired, already in bed, or watching a program that I would not interfere with. This is frustrating; however, I work it all out in the end.

Chapter 8: Dating and Intimacy

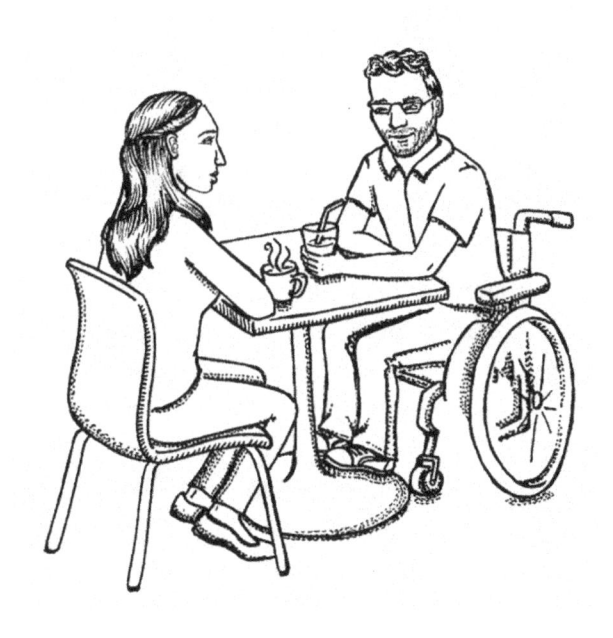

What It's Like to Date with CP

Since I had not yet found myself in a monogamous relationship through high school, college or meeting through friends, I decided to try another route. In 2012, at the age of twenty-three, I signed myself up for online dating — another word for "On The Market." Believe it or not, I've spoken to roughly 1,200 girls, and that's not counting the ones I met in high school.

Knowing my situation, I thought being open and honest was the right thing to do, even though I knew it wasn't going to be an easy road. The online profile I created outlined my personality and what I've been looking for in a relationship, and ends with "be willing to look past whatever physical limitations that I might have to see what I can offer her from my heart. A common area would be understanding what it is to be disabled and a willingness to learn more about cerebral palsy. However, the greatest element would be the willingness to learn and want to understand what truly beats within my heart."

Fears, Frustrations and Future

One of my biggest relationship fears is that my partner could leave me for an able-bodied person. I mean it could happen to anyone and it has, right? However, I'm at a higher risk than most guys because I require a bit more care. I'm not being pessimistic harbouring that kind of outlook; I think I'm just being real. This is probably how most disabled people feel or they have at least thought about it as a possibility.

In my experience, some of the girls I've crossed paths with have been willing to date men who are self-centred, prone to cheating, immature and generally scummy. I'm not sure why women would be with someone who treats them so poorly. I also shake my head in wonder when someone thinks they can change their partner into what they want or to rid those partners of their more unsavoury personality traits. Perhaps these women are content with the superficial things for the short term, and while they may not see the relationship going long term, maybe it is good enough until something better comes along.

When girls say, "I don't think I can be that woman for you, but I know one day you will find that special lady," or when they ask if we can still be "friends," I've always felt like that was them clearing their conscience so they could stop communicating with me. I'm not the type of guy who wants to remain friends with someone from a dating site. That's not why either of us is there. If you don't like my personality, I get that, but don't use my disability as an excuse for not being able to fall in love with me.

I've noticed that the older I get, the more understanding women become, but it's still not enough. I understand that when we're young, we're immature and selfish, so dating someone with a physical disability isn't something most kids would want to contend with. There's no doubt in my mind that girls find my personality attractive. Most of them claim to be fine with the fact that I have CP, but they're always scared of what the future would look like in terms of caring for me and herself, having children, and life in general. And I totally get that. They are the consequences of my life, but it's how you adapt that's important. I always look for ways to make things work, but sometimes finding that answer isn't easy.

Another obstacle I face when finding a partner is having to work with my physical needs. Trust me, I totally get it. I'm not going to lie, I wish I could provide more physically. Cook, drive, be the handyman, cut the grass and all the other things involved with being a husband. And with that being said, it doesn't mean I can't do anything. I can definitely help out. I want people to know that I'm not looking for a caregiver. I'm looking for the love of my life. Yes, I know that I need assistance with feeding, toileting, bathing and dressing, but think about it this way, it's no different than having your significant other share a romantic moment with you, giving you a piece of something on her plate or joining you in the bath/shower — *oops, that's way too much info.* However, I strongly agree that I should have a personal support worker in the mornings during the week, depending on our day-to-day routine. After all, I think it's only fair for my significant other to focus on getting herself ready to take on the day.

"Refuse to worry about tomorrow, but deal with each challenge that comes your way, one day at a time. Tomorrow will take care of itself." (Matthew 6:34, TPT)

My Experience with the Online Dating World

So, I decided to take a step and try to meet someone online. I was excited and nervous at the same time. Excited — to see what was out there and if there was a special woman waiting for me. Nervous — because of my past experiences and knowing that my CP was the big factor. I started with Match, knowing that there would be more girls looking for something serious — well, you'd hope — and Plenty of Fish — well, you never know. That's where my cousin met his wife and some people found each other. In 2015, I thought I would give eHarmony a try, since it's similar to Match. In 2019 and 2020, I signed up on Tinder, Bumble and Hinge, but it still comes down to the same thing over and over. I have CP and it's not desirable. It's devastating most days to live with rejection when I know I deserve happiness and intimacy — *I deserve better, period.*

After a few months of messaging people, I noticed that I wasn't receiving any responses back but knew my messages were read. At that point, I decided to remove the part about having CP to see if that would change anything. Sure enough, I started receiving messages the following week. Once we began talking and learning more about our personalities, drive, hobbies, future goals and what we wanted in life, I would open up and explain that I was born with a physical disability. As expected, things started to deteriorate after that revelation either right on the spot or within weeks. Over the years, I have switched back and forth disclosing my physical disability, and even when it states on my profile not all girls read it. "Damned if you do, damned if you don't."

Another obstacle I face is employment. Luckily and thankfully, I do have an education under my belt. However, the most frequently asked questions are "Do you work? Where do you work, or what are your work hours?" It puts me in a difficult position in terms of what to say. It makes me wonder if they view me as this lazy guy who's useless but travels the world or just doesn't care. This is when I explain my situation. Some understand, while others don't.

I want to show you some of the things that have been said to me over the years to help illustrate my point. Things that have got my hopes up only to bring them crashing back down in the end.

- "Omg, I'm so sorry. That's amazing how you pushed yourself all this time to overcome CP."
- "Sorry to hear about cerebral palsy but I'm impressed that you haven't let it define you or stop you. Is that something that can get worse? Glad to hear that and your positivity is inspiring."

Dating and Intimacy

- "I'm sorry I've been distant the last few days, but to be honest, I needed some time to think. Getting to know you has been wonderful so far. I feel as though I am not as strong of a person as I thought. I'm having a hard time with some of the things you have shared with me. I feel like an awful person but I need to be honest with you, that is the fair thing to do. I feel like we are meant to be friends, God has put you here in my life for many reasons I'm sure. I do believe also because I really do need someone like you to talk to a lot of the time. I'm sorry, I feel like any way I say that it will hurt you and that's not what I want at all. I truly hope that you will still want to talk to me as a friend."
- "My life right now feels like such a mess. The biggest thing that is attracting me to you is your positivity. Your amazing, beautiful outlook on life."
- "Wow, this is a lot to take in. I wasn't expecting this. I'm not a shallow person but I'm not sure at this point you would be able to offer me everything I'm looking for in a serious long-term relationship. I apologize for my ignorance but you said you depend on people to look after your physical needs. I am not prepared at this point in my life to be a caregiver to my 'husband' because that is my goal on this site is to find someone to love, marry and start a family with. I apologize and I feel terrible but like I said before, I want someone that is going to be able to be my equal in every way."
- "You seem too good to be true?! How has someone not snatched you up?"
- "What caught my eye was you are smiling in every picture and your profile said that you were social and liked new adventures. I feel like your pictures showed off your personality which I liked."
- "Wow, that's really amazing that you have such a great outlook on life and know exactly what you want."
- "I don't mind us texting and even getting together. I just want us both to be realistic that with my schedule I can not make it to Hamilton often so something long term between us is not likely. I think you're smart and kind and you're a great guy!"

- "I'll still like you for you, your personality and your big heart. Your CP changes nothing. Your joy for life inspires me, you have a kind heart and a killer smile. I appreciate how you put family first. As much as you're an amazing guy, I don't know if I could handle it in the long run in regards to meeting your needs properly and my mental health. I wish you luck, I know there's someone out there for you."
- "It's just that I have a super active lifestyle and I'd like to be with someone who's just as active as I am. I'm looking for someone who can play sports with me and travel frequently."

As you can see, girls are interested in the beginning but reel back as soon as they find out about my disability. A lot of them are very honest about their feelings, but most of them just disappear immediately, not wanting to deal with any of it. If your partner had an accident, would you leave them on the spot? I have seen a good handful of couples that have had this happen and I'm always happy to see them move on together despite having to overcome their new reality. I just want everyone to put themselves in my shoes and imagine what it would feel like to be able-bodied for most of your life only to become disabled one day. What would you do? How would you feel if people treated you as less than human? Would you like feeling invisible and overlooked?

Another thing that I find interesting is when girls tell me how important faith is to them and claim to attend church every week; I find it rude and ironic that they would dismiss me after hearing about my disability. They just throw me away like garbage. I'm being honest with them, but they show their true colours in the end. It's hypocritical to manipulate your faith to fit your own desires and selfishness. Jesus said, "We are all equal and all of us are loved by God. We all have a purpose. We are created for God's great purpose."

I'm not ashamed of myself or the role that I have been given from God. However, online dating has been hard for me. Every single time I get turned away, I just want to give up. I'm always second-guessing or intimidated with the next girl I talk to because I know what the outcome is going to be. If I could be myself and not worry about my disability, I know I would be in a relationship by now. Out of all the girls I talked to or went on a date with, I would say a good handful felt like we could work. The rest of them were self-absorbed or had some sort of mental issue — no joke — but I still move forward because I simply won't give up. I will admit that it took me a while to get that negative feeling out of my head before I truly realized and understood that it wasn't me. Everyone who rejected me wasn't my loss, it was theirs. However, I believe that God is granting me a favour by not moving forward with them. He is preparing me for a special woman.

Disabled or not, I still love the life I'm living. However, it saddens me how it has taken away so much from me like finding someone special to love. Most girls absolutely love my personality and sense of humour (I mean who wouldn't?!) but it's my physical limitations that put them off. When you're told, "You're what a man should be," or "You're the most genuine guy I know," it's obvious that it's not who I am as a person that's stopping them from wanting to take things further.

Would a Disability Site Be Any Easier?

In 2018, I signed up for a disability site. A few people have suggested that I expand my horizons and see if there's anyone out there who would truly understand what it's like to live with a disability by finding someone who actually has one herself. With that being said, would I date a woman who has a physical disability? Absolutely. We need to have a connection, but yes, I would. I was on the disability site for a month and my experience was less than successful compared to the regular dating sites I use. Only one woman responded, although there aren't many in the area; I knew something wasn't right with her and decided not to pursue it.

During my online adventures, I've also experienced some very strange "girls" who were spammers or people using fake photos to try to guilt you into sending money. Lots of people say their parents are sick or their brother is dead so they need some help. This was especially prevalent on the disability dating site, perhaps because people with disabilities are the most vulnerable and exploitable. It's sick and disgusting that people would do this to others. I'm obviously too smart for these schemes, so I often play along by asking personal questions like, "What hospital is your mom at and who's the doctor looking after them?" Asking them to do video chat is another way to get them pissed off too, but they just take off once they've been found out. There are a lot of sick people in this world.

First Online Date

After two years of online dating, I finally got a date in June 2014. She was from out of town and worked with special needs as an educational assistant. She drove to Hamilton, which was about half an hour away from her. I really appreciated her driving that distance to meet someone she had never met before. If I was able to drive myself, I would have driven there and I am sure my dad, brother, cousin or a friend would have taken me too. However, I wanted to be independent and have some privacy instead of being chaperoned.

We met at a strip plaza near me; we shared tons of stories, a variety of conversations and laughs, and we got along well. I was amazed by how easily she understood my speech after just meeting for the first time. She wanted to go on another date after that one. We both tried setting another one up, but it just wasn't working out. After a few weeks, we tried again but eventually grew apart.

I Just Wasn't What She Was Looking For....

For several months, I had been talking to this girl online who seemed to be really nice. We got on really well and talking to each other seemed easy. She lived over an hour away from me but was studying at McMaster University, not far from my house. We would text daily but never had a chance to meet. I took my time telling her about my physical disability because I wanted someone to have a chance to know me first before making any judgments. She completely understood why I took my time when I eventually told her.

She suggested we go to the movies. I thought, "Our first date is a movie date?" It's not the first date I would have liked to choose, but I didn't make a fuss. After the date, she texted me to say that she had a good time and would like to do it again sometime. We continued to talk daily and I tried setting up another date. She always had an excuse for not being able to make it, but still talked to me until I confronted her about whether she was serious or not. She then claimed to only have an interest in dating non-white guys. We obviously never spoke again.

A Most Awkward Date

March 2017, I had been communicating with this local girl for about a month. We seemed to get along well and had the similar interests. Before we started to have conversations, I was upfront and honest with her about my CP. I didn't want to deal with it later on in our friendship. She told me it wasn't an issue and that it wouldn't change anything. "You are who you are. I don't judge or anything," she told me. "You seem like an amazing person and I'm willing to get to know you more regardless of what you have or don't have." She wanted to meet and went on to say that "I was a catch" and "was the full package."

We met at Starbucks, and I have to say that it was the most uncomfortable, weird and strange date I've ever been on. I felt like she lied about who she was and I had told her everything about me. The date lasted not even half an hour and I did most of the talking. She was shy, uncomfortable and the way she present herself wasn't going to work with me.

Dating Woes

I was chatting with this very sweet and understanding girl for the previous four months before we decided to meet. Prior to our date, we communicated daily and had great conversations.

Once I got to know her sweet, uplifting, happy personality and she got to know mine, I asked if she could read my profile, specifically the part where I talk about having a physical disability, because up until that point we hadn't discussed it.

"Yes, I did read your profile because you seemed eager about it," she said.

"Well, it's not that I was eager about it. I just don't think it's right and fair for you not to know before we met," I told her.

"You have a very positive attitude and outlook on life," she observed. "You know what you want and what you're looking for and I did read about your physical disability. I would never judge. One of my closest guy friends has a physical disability."

Even though I have liked most of the girls I talked to and met a dozen, I really felt that there was a unique connection with this one. She offered to pick me up for our date, which I felt was very caring and understanding. But for the first date, I didn't want her to go out of her way.

Our date was on a Tuesday afternoon in August at a Starbucks. We shared lots of stories, a variety of conversations and laughs, and got along really well for two hours, including taking a walk through the mall. "I can drive you home," she offered after the date. I told her that my mom was across the street at my dad's hair salon waiting, but thanked her for the offer. "Can I meet her?" she asked, which I thought was very sweet of her. She did end up meeting my mom that day.

We continued to chat after our date. I waited for a few weeks until I asked her for a second date and suggested dinner or a movie. She said, "To be honest, I'm not a fan of movies. I rarely watch them and I fall asleep inside movie theatres. I'm sorry!" At the time, I was thinking to myself it didn't have to be a movie; it could be whatever she wanted. She mentioned saving up dessert coupons at a restaurant so I suggested that as an alternative, but nothing came of it.

We would check in weekly to talk about our week and upcoming events, but I knew I wasn't going to get a second date with her. I really liked her and she would still text me. She said she works a lot, so I wanted to be patient with her when she wouldn't give me a straight answer. After several months of not getting anywhere with her, I asked her one more time if she wanted to go out? This would have been the sixth time since our first date. Finally, she answered my question the way I was expecting her to. "I'm not opposed to hanging out, but truthfully, I have no spare time. I work two jobs plus baseball twice a week and my boyfriend lives an hour and twenty minutes away. I am not around Hamilton as much in the summer. That was the first I heard about this boyfriend. She couldn't give me a straight answer for months and suddenly uses this as an excuse. I don't know why people can't just be honest instead of stringing people along.

After chatting with another girl who was finally from the Hamilton area, we decided to meet. We seemed to have similar personalities, ambitions and interests, but I didn't tell her I had CP yet. I wanted her to get to know me first before writing me off. She wanted to get together sooner than I was ready to especially since I hadn't filled her in yet. I don't feel right meeting a girl without first being honest and upfront about myself. When I told her, she was understanding and still wanted to meet. We met at another Starbucks because I didn't want to bump into someone I knew or a previous date — how embarrassing would that be? Well, sure enough, I did run into someone. Luckily I was early and was able to chat with him before she came. The guy didn't believe me when I told him I was meeting someone there. She arrived and I bought drinks for us and we began to chat. We held a steady conversation, shared some stories and laughed for an hour and a half. With a hug, we parted ways afterwards.

It was about a week later before I heard anything from her. I had been through this multiple times before so I was expecting all sorts of excuses. "Hi, Kyle. Sorry for the late reply. It's been a bit busy on my end. At the moment, I can't really commit to anything because of my schedule and some other stuff that's going on, so it wouldn't be fair. You seem like a great person and I hope you find what you're looking for. Take care." And just like that, another person made their exit.

I'm not saying this to make myself look good or to put other guys down, but girls often tell me things like I'm easy to talk to, I say all the right things, I know what I want in life. I'm a very happy, positive guy in my photos and I look like fun. Everyone in my life knows this about me already. I know this! Yet, I'm always left in the dust after they see me in person. I think it shows you that I should have been in a relationship by now if it weren't for my disability.

The Worst Date I've Ever Been On

I decided to try the dating app Tinder to see who else was out there. I was actually getting some bites. I started chatting with a girl who recently moved to Hamilton from the Cambridge area. I'm an open-minded person, but I also know what type of woman I'm looking for and what will fit with my personality, family and friends.

We chatted quite a bit and, within a week, she kept insisting on meeting, which I felt was too soon. I agreed to meet with her so she would stop asking. Prior to the date, some of the things that she was telling me were a bit concerning.

"Connecting with people and making friends isn't easy for me to do," she told me through chat one day. "I guess because I'm quiet and people think I'm not nice or something so they ignore me." She continued to say that nobody really hangs out with her and that she didn't get along with her family.

I didn't think she was going to be a good fit for my personality or my lifestyle. Then she eventually told me that she had Asperger's. I met with her to give her a chance because even though it's a different situation than mine, I know what it's like.

We met at Starbucks on a beautiful afternoon and I offered to buy her a drink, but she declined. Unfortunately, the date only lasted about twenty minutes. She had an attitude and could not engage in conversation. I had to pull words out from her and come up with questions to get the conversation going. She just sat there with this miserable look on her face. This was by far the worst date I had been on other than one from a few years ago. Even though I knew that she wasn't for me, I didn't want to back out and look like a jerk; I wanted to give her a chance. I felt so bad and awkward and for the first time in my life, I had to tell her that I was sorry and this wasn't going to work. She just got up and left without so much as a goodbye.

Hey, I Know You!

I'm constantly chatting with girls from dating sites. Always meeting new ones a few times a week, give or take. I found this sweet and understanding young woman who is from Hamilton, which was a bonus. After chatting daily for two months, we discovered that we had so many things in common and I loved talking and laughing with her, even if we disagreed on hockey teams — thankfully, she wasn't a Bruins fan because that would have been the end of it. At some point in our many conversations, we discovered that we went to the same high school.

She found her high school yearbooks at some point and looked through them. "I believe we are in a picture together," she told me one day. "The girls' softball team picture. I think it's you. It looks like you. I played on the baseball team and you're in the picture."

I laughed and texted, "Didn't I tell you that you should know me?"

"You did and I apologize for not remembering a grade eleven softball team picture from too many years ago," she responded. "However, I don't recall you saying anything about you knowing me either!"

"There's no need to apologize," I responded back. "I didn't even know that or think about looking through the yearbook. We're both even and I'm flattered that you don't remember me. I also had blonde hair in grade nine then when I went back to my natural colour with curly hair."

I was super surprised that she didn't recognize me since I was popular and stood out more than an average student. After she got to know more of my charming personality, I asked if she recalled "a cute guy with an infectious smile and always well-styled hair, speeding around the hallways with his power wheelchair." After she still didn't recall, I told her about my physical disability. A few people suggested being upfront with people about my CP, which I did try but felt like it wasn't working for me. I do say in my profile that I have physical challenges that won't hold me back from being the man I dreamed to be.

When I told her, she said that my disability didn't change anything for her. "I try to be an understanding person and not judge what someone can or can't do. The character of a person is much more important to me than anything else. You seem to be a great guy (with many special 'gifts') and don't let life's challenges hold you back. I'll be honest and say I know very little about CP or the different types so you may have to teach me. Up until now I have thoroughly enjoyed talking to you and hope that it can continue," she told me. "You have been so sweet, kind and caring as well as keeping me laughing and smiling the whole time, even with you being ridiculous and reading my mind at times."

We agreed to meet... again, but this time we actually knew each other. We met on a cold Saturday evening at Starbucks. The place was super busy, which I couldn't believe at the time, but I guess people need their fix. This date was actually one of the best and longest I've been on. It was four hours of non-stop laughs and conversation. However, as usual, I got a text a few weeks later effectively ending the relationship.

"I've been doing some thinking and I'm not being fair to you," she wrote to me. "You are such a great guy and I have thoroughly enjoyed every minute of talking and getting to know you, but, unfortunately, I think it would be best for us to only be friends. I'm so sorry, this is all on me and I don't want to hold you back from finding someone special. We have so many things in common and I love talking and laughing with you, even if we disagree on hockey teams. I would love to be friends, however, I completely understand if that's not something you are interested in." I really wasn't, but I told her about the book I was writing and let her know that I might write about our experience in the book. She let me know that she would read my book when it was published and she hoped I would become a famous author. "I know that special person for you is out there and you have no idea how sorry I am that it's not me."

Intimacy Is Just Out of Reach

Sex is a topic that evokes a lot of feelings and thoughts for me and I've been reluctant to write about it. However, I think I should because after all, it can be an important and normal aspect of everyone's lives.

I associate sex with polarizing emotions like happiness and sadness, fear and joy, and insecurity and actual intimacy. These thoughts and emotions aren't mutually exclusive to people with disabilities either. For those who have it, there's nothing better. For those who don't, there's nothing worse.

I know that I've accomplished a lot over the years; however, I'm always worrying about my future. To be exact, I worry about marriage and sex. I'm more troubled by sex than marriage and worry that I'll never experience it in my lifetime. In my mind, this is a totally legitimate concern and one that I have no clear answer to; all I have is hope. Relationships, in general, have been such a big obstacle for me growing up because the girls I met weren't interested in being with someone who has CP. So, I've been at a huge disadvantage from the start.

Over the years, I've been asked insensitive questions like: "Can I have sex and does it work down there?" After a handful of times, I had enough and decided to strike back by asking, "Does your vagina work?" Of course, that never went over well, but I'm sure they got the point. Maybe they don't think it's rude to ask someone with a disability or simply do not know, but in reality, it is especially the case when you don't know the person very well. Just think of how it makes that person feel to be asked such a thing point-blank.

We explore the myth that one has to have a certain body type in order to attract a sexual partner and to experience sexual pleasure. Once again, not only does a disabled person see able-bodied people having sex but these people are always stereo-typically slender, muscular attractive bodies. It makes people whose bodies are less than perfect wonder if they are desirable in any way. It makes them pessimistic about finding love and may give up over time. It isn't true that a perfect body brings someone perfect love any more than a perfect table setting promises a delicious meal for reasons that are a mystery. Humans' bodies come in all shapes, sizes and abilities. We are not all made in the same mould and instead of celebrating differences, people with disabilities may suffer from a negative body image. Everyone is vulnerable to seek for love and pleasure that we want to attain some imagined level of physical perfection.

It's not about being positive or having faith. It's about the experience and not carrying around the pressure. Now, I know it sounds like I'm worried about what other people think. Honestly, I couldn't care less because I'm responsible for only myself and nobody else. I understand that I'm in a difficult situation where I'm basically trapped. Who would want to have sex with me? Would I be able to satisfy my partner? It's hard to admit this, but I've convinced myself on some level that I've already had sex to help with the psychological stigma that's attached to being a "virgin." I'm lying to myself on the inside so I don't feel the pain. If I was given the opportunity, I wouldn't have to carry around all this pressure I feel every day.

I'm not saying if my situation were different, I would take advantage of a girl just to have sex. Absolutely not. I'm not that type of person. If I was in a serious relationship and we both loved and trusted one another, then yes, but only if she's okay with it.

Several years back, I was talking to my dad about what I was going through and my feelings about sex. He made me realize that none of this was my fault. I understood what he meant by that. It meant that "I'm trapped" and wasn't given a choice in the matter. I have always been the type of guy who feels relieved after I've done something for the first time, as the pressure of not having done something finally gets lifted. The stigma of being a virgin is the most devastating part because society and the media glorify sex. You feel like if you're not doing it, you're nothing and probably the only person in the world who isn't.

Of course, my hope is to find a special woman who will want to be intimate with me, and someone who can be my first and last. But how long should someone wait for such a romantic thing to happen before looking elsewhere? I feel like my situation is incredibly unfair and everyone regardless of their circumstances is entitled to intimacy.

Over the last couple of years, some friends, my cousin and I have researched and contacted different organizations that specialize in intimacy issues with disabled people, also known as sexual surrogacy. These organizations understand what I'm going through and help a lot of disabled people experience intimacy in a safe and trusting environment. The problem is nothing like that exists in Ontario. British Columbia is the main base of operations for Canada, with a whole bunch of places across the border in the States. So far nothing has panned out because I would have to travel, which could be expensive, for the possibility of an experience.

Some of you may disagree with me and say wait until the right person comes along. But just think about that for a moment and remember everything I've written about in this book. I've done everything in my power to be in a relationship for years and it's becoming more apparent that I need to explore other options. If you were in this situation, what would you do? How would you feel?

I still fight and pray for a better tomorrow and I will never let my CP stop me from doing what I want to do. I will live the life God gave me and I know he has made me a stronger and better person.

Dating and Intimacy

Having a Family of My Own

Most people try to understand the experiences I go through, but nobody truly understands the dynamic aspects of it. At most, we intend to understand and empathize with someone's challenges emotionally, physically, and psychologically. However, do we ever know what others go through?

I haven't yet experienced a lot of things that I would like to do and to have. But I can honestly say that I can only imagine what others aren't able to experience because some of life's pleasures are not accessible to me.

I am extremely proud of and grateful for my closest friends and cousins, *especially male friends and cousins* who have taken the role of a gentleman, husband and father, giving their love, respect, interests and responsibility. These role models have my absolute respect and support. That's how it should be.

What I don't have respect for are men who don't take responsibility, who don't grow up and take the next step of being accountable. This also goes for women because it's not just men. I also have zero tolerance for a father or mother who doesn't take full responsibility for taking care of and interacting with their kids. It makes me angry because I would love to have a child of my own. I would never do that to my own or someone else's children.

For as long as I can remember, I've always hoped to have children of my own. I know that my mobility has decreased over the years, so I struggle with one question: is it selfish of me to keep dreaming about love and having a family?

I've asked myself another question that I'm often asked by woman I'm chatting with: whether I think having children would be a challenge for me. I would be lying if I said "No." I know it would be hard, but I would make it work because that's the kind of person I am.

I know it would be a challenge in various ways during the infant to early toddler stages because of the level of hands-on tasks that are required. The feeding, changing and the never-ending list of tasks would mostly need to be done without my assistance, but I would make sure to help out and be present in any way I physically could. Once my children are past that stage, it would be a lot easier because I could start handling them and they would start to understand me through my speech articulation issues. Whenever I see a father interact with their children — such as pushing them in a buggy/wagon, playing at the park or doing sports with them, and so forth — I often play over that thought on my mind of, "How am I going to interact/do these things with my own children?" I guess it doesn't take into account what the children would be like personality-wise, but again, it's something we could work through and manage.

What Am I Looking For in a Woman?

I have always been searching for that woman who would be perfect for me. Someone to love and respect. She must be fun-loving, as I am a goofy, silly guy who loves to have a great time. Someone who will be my best friend, whom I can't wait to come home to. Someone whom I can spend my life with and grow old with. Someone whom I can wake up every morning with and bring each other joy. Go to sleep each night knowing that she loves me for being me. And of course, someone to laugh and tease.

I'm trustworthy, honest, sincere and enjoy deep meaningful conversations. Having someone to share dreams, our thoughts or just daily events with is very important to me. These are important traits and attributes I look for in a partner. Also, I truly hope I will have a chance to have children of my own, the pleasure of being a father and, of course, the pleasure of being a husband.

I am hoping the universe will lead me to the love of my life, to share our hopes and dreams together; even though I have physical challenges, it doesn't nor will ever hold me back from being the man I dream to be.

I will admit that when I was younger and started asking girls out, I would let myself down and feel that it was my fault for having CP. However, as I've grown older and understand more, I realize that it isn't my fault because I was made for a specific reason by God.

Despite my frustrations, I believe there is an absolute, perfect woman waiting for me. I know that one day I will find someone who will cherish every second of our time together because of my genuine heart and personality. Having CP has made me a stronger and better person, but it's my love, care, humour and emotion that I want to be known for.

Dating and Intimacy

As I share some of my experiences with dating, I know that relationships and even marriages have their ups and downs without having to contend with CP or any other disability. Many different reasons can factor into breakups and divorces. Some of us are lucky to find their true love, while others have a few relationships before they find that special one.

I may or may never find my soulmate, but I can strengthen my relationship with good friends and family. And I might never have children of my own, but I find great joy in watching my friends' and cousins' children grow.

There are people who have never been married or have kids but will be very involved with their brothers', sisters' or friends' lives and their children. It's about whether you want to put yourself into their lives and make the effort.

One of the things that helped me over the years is being surrounded by my family and friends, especially in the last five years when my cousins and friends, true friends, were getting married and starting a family. When my cousin Matthew and his wife Ashley had their first daughter Millisle (Millie) in 2017, I took on the role of being that "fun" cousin. And in that same year, my good friend Steven from college and his wife Nikki had their first son Charlie in 2017, and later a daughter Scarlett in 2020. I take so much delight in my role as "Funcle" Kyle to Charlie and Scarlett. In 2021, my cousin Jeff and his wife Erika had their first son Logan. Logan was born a week after my birthday. It would have been sweet to share the same birthdays. I guess Logan wanted his own birthday and I don't blame him. However, if he was born on May 9th, he would have received $1,000 from me for sharing the same birthdays — *Logan will regret this when he finds out*. December 2021, my long-time friend James and his wife Sarah will welcome their first child. There will finally be a little Wombat running around. I'm looking forward to having more nephews and nieces in the future. As you know, I absolutely adore kids and treat my cousins' and friends' children as if they were my own. To all of my nieces, nephews and the children of the next generation, I hope you know that I will always be there for you if you need anything. Sometimes, you just need someone other than your parents to be there for you.

I completely understand that I don't stand alone in this world in terms of being single, wanting to be married or starting a family of my own; it isn't the end of the world, and it doesn't mean I need to give up. I've always been a warrior and have the same desires as everyone else. Having children of my own would be amazing, but it's a special gift to have one of God's children.

My advice for everyone is to never stop looking or give up on finding someone special — *she or he is out there!*

Chapter 9: My Faith and Spirituality

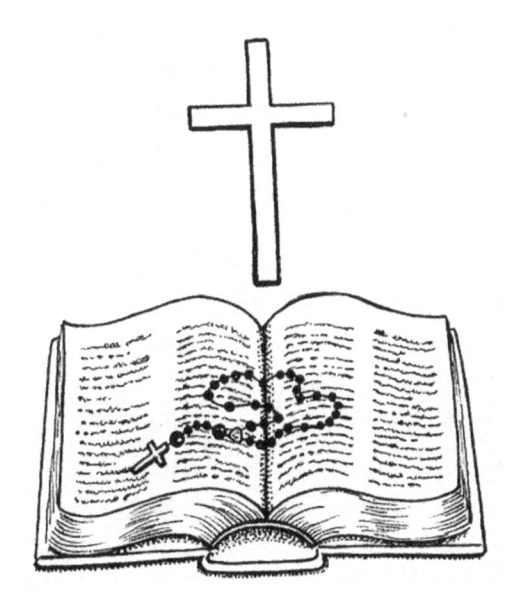

My Faith Is a Journey of Gratitude

More recently, I read Biblical scripture in Psalm 139:16 TPT: "You saw who you created me to be before I became me! Before I'd ever seen the light of day, the number of days you planned for me were already recorded in your book." This significantly touched me to know that the God of Abraham,

Isaac and Jacob wrote a book about each one of His creation in Heaven before any of us was born. Belief in the Bible remains a personal choice and in faith, I believe that all Biblical scripture is the Word of God, inspired by the Holy Spirit. I have since come to understand that my book in Heaven reveals God's will for my life.

Christian evangelist John Bevere, elaborates further on this scripture in the article "There's a Book in Heaven About You," stating, *"God wrote a book about you before your parents even thought of having you — before a single day had passed. Celebrities and rulers aren't the only ones with books containing their life stories. No, yours is recorded too, and the amazing reality is this: it was mapped out and penned by God before you were born. You may protest, 'But my life has had bumps, bruises, and even wrecks due to my bad choices. Did God author that?'"*

No! God mapped out our lives, but it is up to us to walk the exhilarating path He created for us. Wrong choices can detour us — but don't be discouraged or condemned. When we stray from the course, genuine repentance can right the ship.

In reflecting on the scripture referenced earlier, I have asked myself if having CP is part of my book that God has written or was it a fluke? I honestly don't think it was God's intention to put me in this situation, but there are positive things that came out of this. God gave me life against all odds because He knows that I am strong enough to move forward and use the special gifts that He has given me.

No, I didn't make any bad choices to deserve any of this; however, it is hard not to wonder why this happened to me. I believe God is a loving Father who does not cause us illness, sickness or disease; rather it all comes back to the fact that we live in a fallen world. Since the sin of Adam and Eve, the perfect state of God's creation throughout the generations has been in decline not only morally, but genetically, as well. Who knows — did the doctors or nurses in the delivery room during my birth made an error? I believe that God made me in His perfect image and designed a path in my life uniquely for me, just like He did for you! God mapped out our lives, but it is up to us to walk in the path He intends for us. I ask the Holy Spirit in prayer that He bless me with revelation knowledge to know God's will in my life so I stay on His course for me. If you believe in God,

My Faith and Spirituality

His Son Jesus Christ and The Holy Spirit, even if you should stray, with a repentant heart we can ask for forgiveness and God, who has no limits, can make things right for you.

You may again question, "But I've had terrible things happen that were not the result of bad choices. Life has dealt me some hard blows. Did God author the disappointments and hardships?"

I believe God wants what is best for us, which may not be what we want, because He is omniscient. God gave us the gift of "free choice" and with that free gift comes the responsibility for us to choose correctly. His will is that we accept His Son Jesus Christ as our Lord and Saviour. Once we do, God infills us with the gift of the Holy Spirit to help us live righteously. Only with the Holy Spirit's help can we discern between good and evil. Sin is all around us and the fallen angel wants mankind to fall like he did and he seeks to steal, kill and destroy us. Consequently, Jesus said we would have tribulation and would suffer adversity just as He did while He was on Earth. The good news is that because God knew what manner of evil would try to overtake you before you were born, He offers His Son as His greatest gift. It's God's will that we say yes and receive Christ. This is what He designed for each of us in our book, and our written days include the right paths for us to walk to stay on course. The Bible in Ephesians chapter 6 reveals that He equips us with the armour of God to combat evil, knowing what each would surely face. In Him we are triumphant. That is why He calls us "overcomers" in His Word.

God knows us better than we know ourselves. He chooses certain people to go through certain challenges because he knows what each can handle. Overcoming these tests builds our character and matures us in faith so we are strong warriors for His will as a result of surviving them.

> "I can do all things through Christ who strengthens me."
> (Philippians 4:13)

I have such a strong, uplifting faith in myself because of all the love and support I receive from my parents, family, friends and the educational system. As I was raised in the Catholic community at a very young age, but old enough to understand the difference between right and wrong, I wondered why God chose to make me, and not someone else, face these challenges? I would pray and pray, hoping that I would be healed or "fixed" by Jesus and God. I realized that nothing was going to change. God knew I wasn't seeing the big picture here.

One of the scriptures that stood out to me is Matthew 9:1-8, TPT Forgiveness and Healing, which says,

> 1: *Jesus got into the boat and returned to what was considered his hometown, Capernaum. 2: Just then some people brought a paraplegic man to him, lying on a sleeping mat. When Jesus perceived the strong faith within their hearts, he said to the paralyzed man, "My son, be encouraged, for your sins have been forgiven." 3: These words prompted some of the religious scholars who were present to think, "Why, that's nothing but blasphemy!" 4: Jesus supernaturally perceived their thoughts, and said to them, "Why do you carry such evil in your hearts? 5: Which is easier to say, 'Your sins are forgiven,' or, 'Stand up and walk!'? 6: But now, to convince you that the Son of Man has been given authority to forgive sins, I say to this man, 'Stand up, pick up your mat, and walk home.'" 7: Immediately the man sprang to his feet and left for home. 8: When the crowds witnessed this miracle, they were awestruck. They shouted praises to God because he had given such authority to human beings.*

As I thought deeper about it, I discovered what his plans were and why he chose me. He created me for a specific purpose and that is to teach the world that nobody is perfect. It's what you do with it and what you want out of it that makes it perfect.

Even going through the bad days, from that point on I knew why God made me for his purpose. I look at it like this: So what? I have cerebral palsy. At least I was given a brain to use and a determination to teach others. My dad always tells me it's a shame that some people who have "It" have no idea what to do with it. That is such a waste of God's gift.

My faith isn't just about God. It's also about everyone around me. I strongly believe if you treat people how you want to be treated — with respect, love, support and laughter — you will be treated that way in return. I'm a people person and can't live without making someone smile and laugh. If I didn't have the love and support from my amazing village, I wouldn't be here today.

I am grateful for my faith and everything that God gave me: a brain to use, determination to teach others, and the love and support from everyone around me.

2020: The World Has Changed Globally

The COVID-19 virus has completely changed the world we live in. What started gaining traction in late 2019 spread rapidly across North America by March 2020. The virus changed many people's lives, socially, physically, mentally and financially. Work, as we knew it pre-COVID, saw forty-hour work weeks; in the months after the worst of COVID, work looks much different. Many people work from home; many industries have had to re-evaluate and adapt their business and workforce, thereby leaving many unemployed or facing a reduction in hours and pay. Essential service has become a common term describing firefighters, police officers, nurses, doctors and even grocery store workers, who are still employed and have had to adapt their styles of work to keep our communities safe.

My family and I had planned to travel to Italy in May 2020 for the first time ever. My mom had been before, but it would have been the first to the rest of us. My uncle Tony and his family were joining us as well and we were all genuinely excited after we finalized a trip that took a year to plan. We were all devastated when we heard about the virus hitting Italy so badly. The virus practically exploded as Italy went into total shutdown after experiencing so many cases and deaths. I was really looking forward to our travels, knowing that it was something my nonna wanted us to do as a family when she was alive. However, it's better to be safe than sorry, so we cancelled our trip, knowing that we would get there one day.

When the government shut down all essential services and told us to stay home as much as possible to reduce the spread of the virus, a lot of us began to panic. It only took a few days for people to start feeling imprisoned. People were seen going through anxiety or complaining about boredom on social media because they hadn't physically socialized with anyone in seven days.

I'm sure the quarantine is a huge adjustment to many people all over the world, but I see it a bit differently. When I listen to people talk about how tragic it is to stay home, I want to just tell them that this is what most people with disabilities go through every day. Most people have had to readjust their lifestyle knowing this would only be temporary or a "new normal" they could live with. Those of us with disabilities don't have that light at the end of the tunnel.

History has shown us that a pandemic is likely to occur every century. It sure seems that way, but we should all be thankful this time around and consider ourselves fortunate enough for the medical advancements, technology and knowledge we've attained in that time period to help us combat COVID-19. We should also be very thankful for all the different ways we can stay connected with our village through social media. As difficult as this global shutdown has been, I've been grateful to spend so much quality time with my family and stay connected without having to cut things short; everyone is only a video call away. I don't even want to imagine what it would have been like to live through this one hundred years ago. However, people still complain because we need to wear masks and must stay confined to our homes where we have food, electricity, running water, WiFi and even Netflix.

The only thing I wish I could have experienced while locked in would be having a significant other by my side and a child of my own (great time to have quality time). I've seen the posts — spouses are driving each other up the wall while being locked in together, but someone like me would jump at the chance to spend so much time together with someone they loved. Some people have been living in quarantine all of their lives. They miss out on social events, always staying in, having no visitors and no social entertainment. I know that I've lived my life patiently waiting for a day where things could be "normal," so think about being stuck in for decades instead of months. Think of how you feel today about the quarantine and expand that to encompass your entire life. It's a heavy thing to think about, isn't it? It is learning to adapt and allowing to except and to move forward and restructure the best that we can. We can put ourselves in survivor mode and make the most of the challenges we face.

My Faith and Spirituality

Everyone wants to achieve certain milestones in life like education, employment, marriage, home ownership, growing a family and so forth. Each milestone can be achieved differently by everyone. Some people achieve all their milestones in appropriate time frames; however, as long as we get there, no matter what road we took or how long it took to get there, we would have considered ourselves successful. Some of us have to wait a little longer due to each person's situation. Although my milestones are few and far between, some I've yet to experience, I can tell you with complete honesty that it's not for lack of trying.

I know there are people around me who have never had a serious relationship and these are people who look like the complete package. But who am I to judge? I just look at them and wonder how that's possible when they can socialize and mingle out in the world. I also wonder how they look at me and if they wonder how they would cope being in my shoes. People do ask me how I cope and face rejection. The simple answer: I won't give up and I won't give in. I live to fight another day because my turn has to be coming soon!

Is COVID-19, the novel coronavirus, a curse or a blessing? I honestly believe that it's both. Here's what many of us know. The outbreak was first identified in Wuhan, China, in December 2019. The World Health Organization declared the outbreak a Public Health Emergency of International Concern on January 30th, 2020, and a pandemic on March 11th, 2020. Many Christians believe this plague was conceived by Satan or man-made to instill fear throughout the world, to cause chaos and economic upheaval as the evil one intends to destroy lives and the world. Although God, who is immutably righteous and just, allowed this to occur, He is using it to further His kingdom. Society and the family unit have been in moral decline with so many marriages ending in divorce, with so much focus on material gain, greed and the "all about me" lifestyle.

However, God turns the tables and he causes good out of evil. With the shutdown, many of us have sought more quiet time with the Lord, in prayer, fellowshipping with family and friends, focusing back on the relationships in our lives, the most important being our relationship with our Lord. He is our great provider and asks that we fear not but surrender our worries to Him. He wants us to live a pure life, a good life and intends for us to share the Good News with others so that more people go to Heaven. He provides for all our needs to live a good life. *"For God has not given us a spirit of fear and timidity, but of power, love, and self-discipline."* (2 Timothy 1:7, NLT)

At the beginning of this pandemic, I think most people came to the realization that a lot of things they enjoyed had been taken away from them and they needed to relearn what it meant to be grateful for what they have in their life. In the end, they had to learn a new appreciation for what they used to take for granted. Realizing what they truly needed to be thankful and grateful for. The world has been slowly opened up on June 19th, 2020, months after the pandemic began, to what is called "the new normal." Although I'm noticing people are turning back to their self-indulgent ways again... sadly enough, which in my opinion will possibly cause a second wave of the virus. On September 28th, Ontario had entered the second wave.

By November 2020, numbers are still climbing. Parts of Toronto had gone into its second lockdown. I feel most people are aware of the seriousness, following the rules of what is asked of us in order to comply with COVID regulations. The vaccination is on its way by the fall of 2021, rumours are now saying as early as the new year, to spring. However, they have stated that most will be able to receive their shot in the late fall.

The first vaccine has been administered to a nurse in Toronto, followed by nurses and staff in long-term care nursing homes. The world is ready to move forward, but we have to be patient and follow the guidelines of our public health and government. The Ontario Government has announced that Hamilton will enter the second lockdown phase for COVID restrictions starting on Dec. 21st. The provincial government's restrictions are set to be in place for a minimum of 28 days. "In Hamilton, the number of cases and hospitalizations are trending upwards and further action is required to help stop the spread of the virus," a statement issued by officials on Dec. 18th said. On Dec 26th, the Premier for Ontario announced another province-wide lockdown, making this the second lockdown in 2020.

On February 16th, 2021, Hamilton was reopened for a few weeks before being placed under COVID-19's grey-lockdown category as of March 29th. Ontario issued another stay-at-home order after being caught up in a third wave primarily caused by more transmissible and deadly COVID-19 variants. On June 11th, the province reopened for the third time and encouraged people to get their vaccinations, in hopes of stopping the spread.

Many are quick to forget once the luxuries and comforts of life are given back. I truly believe we need to learn from this unexpected event because God is trying to teach us to appreciate what we have and to spend time with our families because that's what truly matters.

Count your blessings!

Life Is Just Temporary; There's an Afterlife

Are you afraid to die? Do you believe that life is only temporary and there's an afterlife when we pass on?

I'm not afraid to die and believe in an afterlife. Some people are afraid to die, but I would ask them why? We all have to leave someday, somehow. It's just a matter of *when* and *how*, not *if*. I'm not saying I'm ready to die anytime soon, because I'm still young and have unfinished business; however, when it's my turn I believe I'll be ready. Even though there are days where I question why I'm still alive, I keep telling myself, "Kyle, stay focused. Think about all the things you've accomplished and know that it's only the beginning. Think about the village you've built and how much you're loved and appreciated by everyone. Your day will come!"

I believe that we go through pain and obstacles in our life so that when we finally reach Heaven we can enjoy our existence. We've earned it. You've put in the time and hard work and this is the ultimate reward. There is no reason to be afraid when eternal life awaits you.

I have read and seen movies about near-death experiences — about people who came back from a short-term death, as it were. These people say they've seen Heaven and it's a peaceful and beautiful place.

Everyone has their own image of what Heaven looks like. Everything I would see is what I would wish for. The same for you. What you see is what you wished for. For me, everyone will be younger. God in His wisdom decided that we should be in our prime and looking the best we ever did.

Whew, thank goodness, because I certainly don't want to look like an old geezer in eternity, would you?

You may have read, heard or possibly seen that Heaven is actually an eternal city that the Bible calls "New Jerusalem." It will be spectacular. As a sampling, here is what it will look like according to scripture in Revelation 21:18-19 and 22:1-5, TPT.

> *A river, clear as crystal, will flow from the throne of God and of the Lamb [Jesus] down the middle of the city. On each side of the river, there will be a tree of life, yielding twelve kinds of fruit every month. The streets will be pure gold, like transparent glass. The walls of the city will be adorned with every kind of jewel, emerald, onyx, amethyst, topaz, etc. There will be no need for a sun or moon, and no need for a temple or church. The presence of the Lord will be its light.*

Is this true or is it someone's imagination that has been passed down for centuries? We will never know until it happens. If you have faith and patience, your questions will be answered. It will be worth the wait. However, I don't think it is far from that description. In fact, it's probably accurate. The only thing I know is the colours and visuals of Heaven will be breathtaking and everything will be *FREE — I hope!* However, we will all have to go through Heavenly Court with God where he passes judgment once we cross over.

So, when it's my turn to leave Earth, I just want one year to myself. A year to indulge and do everything I would like to do. In the first six months, I want to see all the people who were in my village and had previously passed on. I want to meet the relatives that I never had the chance to meet, and reconnect with the ones who were taken when I was very young. I also want to finally meet my sister. Yes, my parents had a miscarriage three years after I was born. I've seen a few different psychics who told me about her. The angels named her Elizabeth and she has long blonde hair and blue eyes — finally, someone in the family who takes after my dad. She didn't survive because she had a hole in her heart. Throughout the years, I've had visions of a little girl with long, curly, blonde hair and blue eyes

My Faith and Spirituality

who visits me. Maybe it's her? When I meet my sister, I will give her a nice, big-brother hug, the biggest one she could ever receive.

After spending time with everyone, I would like to make a reservation with God and Jesus so we could have a few glasses of red wine over dinner. Oh yeah, and some Baileys afterwards. I certainly hope that there is Baileys in Heaven; otherwise, I would have to take a trip back to Earth, like Lucifer did, to buy a dozen cases at the LCBO. Although that would mean I would be returning back to Earth more than that one time. I would have to bring the recipe to make my own Baileys back to Heaven because we wouldn't want another fallen angel on God's hands.

After my first six months, I want to do all the things I've wanted to do but couldn't while alive. First, I would no longer have CP. I would feel no pain in my body and wouldn't need help from anyone — with that being said, I'm thankful and beyond appreciative of everyone's help. I want to experience myself and test my own abilities to see what I can actually do.

Even though I can swim, I want to know what it feels like to swim at my own pace. If I decide to swim fast, I can, or slowly so I can take in every sight I see with the heavenly water surrounding my body. As I swim further, I would see the beautiful colours around me and note how easy it is to breathe. I would love to play sports again, in fact, all sports. However, I would like to play hockey on real ice skates to experience what it feels like. Also, I wouldn't mind playing sledge hockey again, but using both of my hands and arms. I would play in the Paralympics since I couldn't in life because I had a "pusher."

Another thing I want to do is run. Yes, I was able to run independently until my hip issues took that mobility away from me; however, I didn't experience what it felt like to truly run. I would feel a tremendous sense of happiness once I've found my rhythm and gained energy, strength, power and accomplishment. I would run forever around a heavenly track, playing my favourite playlist of songs. It would be bliss.

I feel the same about riding a bike, climbing a mountain, skiing and driving a car. Hmm, I'm not too sure if we need to drive in Heaven, but maybe they can make an exception for me and let me take a test drive to get it out of my system. There are so many other things, but I think I have given you the idea. Also, I would love to build a house in Heaven, since I'm an architectural technician after all, completely by myself. I think God can trust me. What's the worst that can happen?

I would love to make homemade Italian food and desserts with Nonna who was always in the kitchen cooking and baking with relatives. Since losing my Nonno at an early age, I would love to reconnect with him and enjoy spending time growing our very own fig tree, making homemade prosciutto, tomato sauce, wine, building things, and playing bocce as he enjoyed all of these things during his time on Earth. In fact, he would most likely help me with the Heaven house I would build.

It would be an honour to play the piano and bagpipes with Grandpa Scott and, of course, play practical jokes on everyone. Playing and singing "Amazing Grace" to Grandma Scott using wind chimes, as she claimed to have heard this song playing on chimes while floating in my uncle George and aunt Jean's pool. I would listen to all the crazy stories she witnessed during her time in Heaven and be amused by the ones on Earth. She would have to tell me all about the things she got herself into since she arrived in Heaven, which I'm sure is plenty.

It would be a dream come true to have a wrestling match with my great-uncle George and other iconic wrestling legends. Washing cars with Uncle Kevin, making sure they were spotless while getting to know him personally since I was only seven years old when he passed. Trying to shoot the puck past my friend, Marc, playing sledge hockey with him as he was an outstanding goaltender. I would spend time talking to Aunt Susan (Susu) about her cats and have a good laugh like we always did. Cousin Claudio who no longer comes for wine and espresso only to have a good laugh again, just like the good old days... and to give him shit for not texting, emailing or calling me back! And my dearest friend Mr. Pizza, who was a true gentleman and a special friend of the family for many years. You will read about these loved ones later in the book.

And, of course, I would love to finally meet and spend time with my sister Elizabeth — or Betty, because that's probably what I would call her. I would love to get to know her personally.

Do you think six months is long enough for all of these requests? If not, I can always ask God for an extension. Oh yeah, I forgot to mention that everyone is welcome to join me, of course. However, you have to be dead and in Heaven before you can keep up with me.

I hope nothing I've written here has gone against anyone's religious beliefs or has ruined their version of Heaven. It's as I said, Heaven will be what you want it to be. I've pictured it in this light and I'm not afraid. I know that I need to keep on the path of goodness and be good to others and myself. Earth is not our final home; we were created for something much better. Your identity is in eternity, and your homeland is Heaven.

Chapter 10: Memories and Celebrations That Will Last a Lifetime

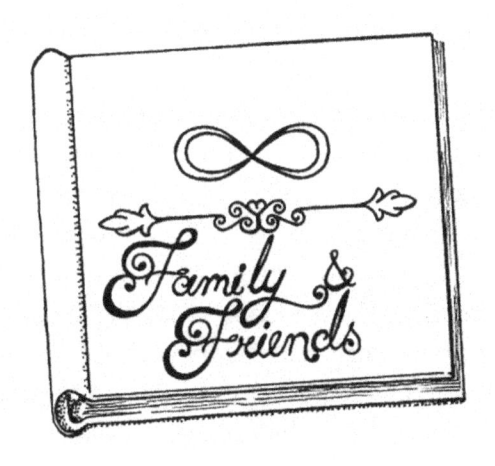

Get Me Back Out There, Coach

From an early age, I've always loved playing sports and my family would always play them with me. One Saturday morning, my aunt Anna and uncle Brian came over for a visit. Every time they visited, Brian and I would play floor hockey, with me playing goalie as usual. However, this time I decided to play a different position. I ended up losing my balance and fell back, right into the corner of an end table. Blood was everywhere because I split my head right open. My mom and aunt rushed to get towels to stop the bleeding, but all I remember saying was that I was totally fine. Their response, of course, was that I needed to go to the hospital. So, off we went to the emergency room to get a few stitches on the back of my head. My mind was only concerned about one thing, though. I asked the doctor who was taking care of me if I could go home and keep playing hockey after this. Obviously, his answer was to refrain from it for a while. What can I say — *I'm a trooper.*

A Disney Wedding Come to Life

The night before my uncle Tony (Fuzzy) and soon-to-be aunt Susan (Suzy) say, "I do," we had a rehearsal at the chapel located at the Old Mill in Toronto, Ontario. My cousin Mark and I were in the wedding party. Mark was one of Tony's groomsmen and I was the ring bearer, and boy, what a handsome little ring bearer I was.

On the wedding day (Saturday, November 22nd, 1997, if I remember correctly), it ended up being a beautiful, clear day with a temperature sitting just below zero. After the ceremony, everyone went to the reception, located in the ballroom straight down the hall. This was the first time I ever experienced a wedding of such a high calibre. The venue had a hill full of trees and gave off an old German vibe — it was like a caption of a scene in *The Sound of Music* when Julie Andrews sings "The Hills Are Alive." The ballroom was beautiful and elegant, full of our family and friends. It had these great-looking French doors that led to a large balcony that overlooked the tree-filled forest area. It really did feel like a movie set.

The snow began to fall ever so slightly that evening when the dancing started, adding a little magic to the event. Tony and his newly-wed wife Susan wanted to go out on the balcony, so they pushed open the French doors and walked out into the snow. Taking care not to slip on the balcony, they began to slowly dance as the snowflakes danced around them. It gently melted on their shoulders and dusted their hair. At that moment, Tony stole the spotlight because of his gorgeous dark black, and now a little less fuzzy, hair. Seeing this was like watching a live-action version of *Beauty and the Beast*.

My uncle Tony and aunt Susan are incredibly special to me. Tony has always been very supportive and involved with my activities since the beginning. He would always play floor hockey in my nonno's and nonna's basement or baseball in the backyard or ballpark. The first time I met Susan was on a warm, sunny day at Ontario Place. When my uncle told me she played hockey and baseball, I thought, "Wow, she's going to be a cool aunt one day." We had many matchups together from that day onward, and I always admired her natural athletic ability.

When the two of them decided to get married, I was super excited for them. I'm surprised I even remember these events being only eight at the time, but it feels just like yesterday to me. I've always been proud of Tony and Susan and even more so since I was a part of their special day.

Hammer Time

On Saturday, May 10th, 2003, I had my Confirmation, which is the sacrament by which Catholics, typically around the age of fourteen, receive a special outpouring of the Holy Spirit. In order to get confirmed, you need to pick a sponsor, usually someone you look up to. I chose my uncle Tony because he always treated me like a son and spent a lot of time playing sports like hockey and baseball with me. Let's not forget all the times he babysat and took me all over the place for outings.

Following the Confirmation, my family gave me a big dinner celebration with our family and friends back at our house. This was a dual celebration because my birthday was the day prior, so this gave us two reasons to celebrate. After everyone arrived and was seated, aunt Susan, was trying to multitask by seating her daughter, Samantha, at the table, and her son, Nicolas, in a high chair. Unfortunately, the tray slipped off the high chair and landed on Grandma Scott's (Evelyn's) hammertoe that she had been dealing with for a while. In an attempt to relieve the pain, she took her shoe off, which was putting a lot of pressure on the toe. She went back to enjoy herself shoeless, thinking the worst was over, but it wasn't.

Mere minutes later, after everyone went back to enjoying each other's company, the high chair tabletop slipped off yet again onto Grandma's toe, but this time she stood straight up, gripping the sides of the dinner table and letting out a yelp of excruciating pain. Most of the people at the table had no idea what happened until they saw blood underneath the table.

My grandpa Walter never missed an opportunity to be sarcastic, especially to his wife. "Well, that fixed your hammertoe," he said.

Still holding the table and dealing with the pain, Grandma shot back, "It's okay for you to say, it's not your toe!" Things were quickly cleaned up and my grandma's toe was looked after as best as possible.

I was thankful to have my family together to celebrate these two special occasions, and even though I wouldn't have forgotten the day to begin with, my grandmother's mishap made it far more memorable. It ended up being yet another prime example of the many, many, many accidents my grandma found herself involved in over the years, which you will discover as you continue reading.

Victimizing Aunt Anna

In April 2006, my aunt Anna and uncle Brian moved in with us while they hunted for a new house. My dad and I love to play pranks on Anna so having her in the house, thankfully for a short period of time, was a dream come true. One night, my dad and I grabbed this large, stuffed monkey and quietly put it beside her pillow. We quietly called her name out until she woke up screaming, only to go back down after whipping the stuffed animal across the room.

The next morning, we asked Anna what the scream was about. With a straight face, she told us it was just a dream. We pushed her some more for something more specific. "A monkey was attacking me!" she shouted, comically loud.

With the empathy of a rock, my dad shook his head and said, "Gee, that must have been awful, Anna."

Another evening, my dad grabbed a mannequin head he owns for hairdressing and dressed it in overalls. We also had arms for some reason and a pair of boots. Knowing that Anna gets up every night to use the washroom, we propped the lifeless and sloppy-looking body on her toilet, adding a little bit of fake blood on the hands for dramatic effect. The entire house was woken at 3:00 a.m. by a blood-curdling scream that night and it was worth every second of lost sleep.

The torture continued almost every night before they moved out. I think all these antics actually gave them the motivation they needed to quickly find a place of their own. My dad and I were sad to see them go. I can't say the feeling was mutual.

Fiftieth Wedding Anniversary

On April 24th, 2009, my grandpa and grandma Scott were celebrating their fiftieth wedding anniversary. We had arranged a small gathering at the La Piazza Allegra Italian restaurant in Hamilton. Their lifetime friends and practically family, Emily and Freddy, happily joined us as well. We ordered different foods off the menu to try a little bit of everything. When the food came, the only sound you could hear was our cutlery clanging together as we stuffed ourselves. Laughter eventually broke the silence because we all realized how much we were enjoying our food.

As we were getting ready to leave, the waitress asked if we needed help getting down a set of five stairs that wasn't far from where we were seated. My dad said to the waitress, "I think we should be okay. I am going to take a few steps back and push, hoping the wheelchair makes a safe landing. Maybe you can stand at the bottom in case something goes wrong?" The look of sheer terror on the waitress's face was priceless.

We all had a wonderful evening that night celebrating my grandparents' Golden Wedding Anniversary. Boy, did my grandma really enjoy the champagne that night.

Pepie the Family Dog

For years, Stirling always wanted a dog. He would always sign out this one dog book from the school library for months at a time. The librarian actually had to stop him one day and prevented him from taking the book out because he basically owned it.

Well, the day finally came, years later mind you, but it came. In September 2009, we adopted a one-year-old Maltese Shih Tzu (also known as a Multi-Shit) named Pepie. When we were looking for a dog, one of my dad's employees at the salon was actually looking for someone to take a dog that her neighbour's daughter left behind when she left for England. The daughter's boyfriend kept the dog for a few weeks before dumping him off at the mother's house.

Pepie and the lady came over to interview us to see if we were the right family for adoption. Pepie is black and white and weighs around twenty pounds. Within half an hour, the lady said, "When would you like to take Pepie?" That night, Pepie became the newest member of our family.

The first couple of months were an adjustment for all of us. It actually took Pepie about half a year to get comfortable with my dad. Our thinking was that the boyfriend mistreated her so she was afraid of men for a long time.

People say that she looks like Pepé Le Pew (the skunk from Looney Toons) and think she is a boy. We would just tell people to think of Pippi Longstocking because she's a girl. She thinks everyone is her friend and loves kids, jumping up to their height to lick their faces. Every single time I'm having a bath, she has to come in and "bathe me" like I'm her little baby. If I'm going to bed or waking up, she has to attack me and wants to play.

Pepie is very affectionate, loving, caring, and has a playful personality. However, she can be stubborn at times — and thus fits right in with the Scott family. She says her prayers each time she eats, morning and night, and won't eat until we've said ours too. Every day she sits down before eating and looks at us until we say, "Thank you God for the food I'm about to eat. Amen," before chowing down. She's also very good at sharing her time with everyone in the house equally and doesn't play favourites.

Pepie has been the absolute perfect dog that anyone could ever ask for and we all love her so much.

Changing Up the D'Agostino Tradition

Traditionally, we celebrated Christmas on Christmas Eve with my mom's side of the family. Long before I was brought into the world, they had large gatherings at one of the relatives' houses, which often had up to forty people. Everybody lived on Locke Street or just around the corner from it, so it made it easy for people to attend. Christmas dinners were always served with lobster and shrimp until someone didn't eat fish and another was actually allergic. The family always attended the Christmas Eve service before opening up their presents with my nonno pretending to be Santa Claus.

At one of our gatherings one year, I started to suspect Santa wasn't really Santa. I was sitting on his lap and noticed that Santa's watch looked familiar. I thought to myself (sorry for the pun), "Wait a minute!" and tried to inspect his face. After a few seconds, I saw right through the disguise and guessed it was my nonno. My dad had a camcorder and taped the whole thing. The funny thing is we had a break-in not long after and someone stole the camera. We were so upset because the tape was still on the camera. We didn't care about the camera itself; we just wished the scoundrel had had the common courtesy to leave the tape behind.

As the family grew and some got married, everyone started a new tradition with more immediate family members, with some of us taking turns to host each year. In 1993, we went to my uncle Joe and aunt Janice's house in Kingston, Ontario. Their house backs out onto a pond, which would freeze, allowing us to put on skates to play some hockey. I was always the goalie. Afterwards, we would come in for a nice Christmas dinner and later do Secret Santa. The remainder of the evening was spent doing puzzles and playing board games.

When my nonno passed away in 1996, Nonna moved in with us three years later. My parents took over hosting Christmas Eve and still continued going up to Kingston on Boxing Day until Nonna passed away.

In 2013, we had decided to try our Christmas gathering in the summertime. My cousin Mark (Joe and Janice's son) was married and living in Ottawa with his son, Daniel. The weather was always bad driving up in the winter and we thought it would be nice for a change. The first year, we met halfway, in Oshawa having lunch at East Side Mario's at a mall, spending a few hours together only to head home the same day.

In 2014, we had dinner at our house on a Saturday night and went to my uncle Tony's on Sunday for breakfast. Uncle Tony and Aunt Susan had bought a new house in Mississauga, so he was excited to host. He wanted to put a pool in the backyard, which would make the gatherings even better. My cousin Mark decided to start a new tradition right then and there by proposing to do the Christmas gatherings in the summer over an entire weekend. That tradition still holds up today.

Nicolas's Confirmation Sponsor

On Thanksgiving in 2014, my cousin Nicolas asked me if I would be his sponsor for his Confirmation. He came up to me with his puppy-dog eyes, all shy to ask. Of course, I said yes. On the day of his Confirmation, I was able to stand behind him while he was confirmed.

We returned to my uncle and aunt's house to celebrate with desserts and to open his gifts. While leaving, Nick thanked me for being his sponsor and gave me a letter that read as follows:

> Dear Kyle,
>
> I am really happy that you agreed to be my sponsor. I hope you will be able to help me with my spiritual needs and guide me in the right direction as I grow older in the church. The reason why I chose you as my sponsor was because I admire and look up to you. You've faced many challenges in your life, however, you are always smiling and make the most of what you have. You are an inspiration to me and inspire me to be a better person.
>
> Love your cousin,
>
> Nick

I was beyond proud of Nick and felt honoured to be a witness for him. When he asked me to be his sponsor, I was touched that not only am I his cousin, but I am an inspiration to him and someone he looks up to. This special event brought back memories of when his dad, my uncle Tony, was my sponsor years before, it's history repeating itself.

Going Down, Down, Down

On Saturday, March 28th, 2015, my uncle Gordon married the love of his life, Theressa. The wedding was held at St. Giles Presbyterian Church in St. Catharines, Ontario. It was a beautiful, clear day with a temperature of -3 degrees Celsius.

Uncle Gordon chose my dad to be the best man and I was the groomsman. they had two of their younger bagpipers, who were part of their Grimsby Pipe Band, Alick and Victoria, pipe the ceremony. After the lovebirds said, "I do," we made our way downstairs to the reception area. My aunt Susan, cousin Brittany and I took the elevator. It was not the standard-looking elevator most of us are used to. It was more of a lift because you had to manually press and hold the button to go up and down. My aunt Susan suffered from anxiety and we were all aware of it. In our family of tormentors, that didn't matter. She was panicking long before we even got on the thing. Brittany reassured her that everything was going to be fine and that it seemed like a sturdy elevator.

As we began to make our descent, Brittany stopped the elevator halfway down.

"What's happening?" Susan screamed.

"Relax. Technical difficulties. It might be weight overload," Brittany teased.

With her anxiety cranked to eleven, Susan belted out, "Oh my God! Get me out of this stupid contraption!"

The Scotts just can't help themselves. Brittany started pushing the buttons up and down to make the lift shake as if it was out of control. Susan started questioning the age of the lift and saying that it was time for it to be laid to rest in the old elevator cemetery. It was obvious that she was catching on, otherwise she wouldn't have started making jokes. The lift made it to the bottom and Susan pushed the doors open to run out. "That blasted thing! Never again!" she said with sweat pouring down her face. Both Brittany and I needed to change our underwear from laughing so hard, but this was payback that was long overdue. Susan was always a mischief-maker, so she completely deserved this.

The wedding reception was small, simple, and attended by close family and friends in the church's gymnasium. The meal was catered by an Italian company, and everyone enjoyed the delicious meal and homemade desserts made by Aunt Theressa, family and friends.

The rest of the evening was easygoing, and open... with a few heartfelt speeches and close company. Everyone was extremely happy for both Gordon and Theressa as they began to start their new life together.

As everyone was leaving that evening, I asked my aunt Susan if she wanted to take another jerky ride on the lift. Straight-faced, she answered, "Heck no!" and stormed up the stairs.

When my uncle Gordon and aunt Theressa received their wedding pictures, we realized that many of the photos had "orbs" in them. Orbs are said to be spirits and ghosts that only a camera can pick up. There was a picture of my deceased grandparents on display at the altar, so we assumed that the orbs were them and that they were present for the event.

My uncle Gordon has been there since my birth. I was told that he waited patiently to see his new niece or nephew before I was born. If I were a boy, I would be the first in the family to carry on the Scott name. We all know that it made him happy to find out he had another nephew.

Our relationship grew over the years and we spent many celebrations together. Who would have ever thought that one day his little nephew would grow up to be a groomsman at his wedding? Being twenty-six at his wedding made me reflect on how fast life can be and how you never know where life might take you. Being a groomsman that day made me so proud.

Aunt Theressa and I had crossed paths since she joined Gordon's pipe band, but it wasn't until the end of 2012 when we officially met. I remember it being a very snowy evening as we were coming home from Kingston. We pulled up to unexpectedly see Gordon shovelling our driveway to welcome us home. He had brought Theressa over to finally meet us. After spending time with her and seeing the love she had for Gordon, I was extremely happy for the both of them. Since then, Theressa and I built a wonderful relationship and have shared many memories together.

Memories and Celebrations That Will Last a Lifetime

The Price is Right

My cousin Jeff and I had started a tradition of going to the Blue Jays games every year. Both Jeff and his girlfriend Erika would give me tickets for my birthday. This year, Erika brought her friend to join us on what I considered to be an incredible day and an all-around awesome experience.

It was August 1st, 2015. The Blue Jays had recently acquired an ace left-handed pitcher named David Price from the Detroit Tigers. He was making his debut that day in the game. Price received a standing ovation when he took to the field. He threw strikeout after strikeout and helped the Jays mount the explosive offensive that they're known for.

Thanks to eleven strikeouts from Price in eight strong innings, his debut led the team to a 5-1 victory against the Minnesota Twins. There were chants of "M-V-P" throughout the crowd that night. The game itself put the Blue Jays in a tie for an American League wildcard spot. The Rogers Centre was sold out on what was a civic holiday with about 45,000 Blue Jay fans and maybe a handful of Twins fans. The Price is Right, as they say!

The Hunt Is Over!

The hunt was over for my good friend Steven. He tied the knot with his wife, Nikki, on Saturday August 15th, 2015, the hottest and most humid summer day at the Amici's Banquet and Conference Centre in Thorold, Ontario. When Steven and Nikki told me while out to lunch one day that they were engaged, I was super excited. I always thought they would make a great "country" couple. Both are like little siblings to me.

Steven and I met in college taking the same course, and he also pushed for a time in sledge hockey. When we first shook hands, I knew we were going to build an incredible friendship that would last a lifetime. When life took us in different directions after college, we kept in touch by going to OHL, AHL and Leafs-Sabres games in Buffalo.

I met Nikki and Steven's mom, Bernadette, for the first time at one of our sledge hockey games in Hamilton. A year later, I ended up meeting Nikki's entire family at an OHL hockey game at Copps Coliseum (now,

FirstOntario Centre) in Hamilton. Nikki's family were very welcoming and were happy to meet me after hearing so much about me. I was overwhelmed by the embrace even though I didn't know the family for very long. They made it feel like I was a part of their actual family.

The wedding ceremony was outdoors under a beautiful wooden pergola surrounded by a colourful garden. Despite the heat, we had a nice on-site band to listen to while trying to stay cool. Each of the wedding parties had their own entrance into the hall. They did a fantastic job including two hilarious entrances, one being Steven's sister Kimberly pulling a groomsman in a little kid wagon with a beer in his hand. Another one saw a re-enactment of the famous scene from *Dirty Dancing* where Patrick Swayze lifted Jennifer Grey in the air, but they switched it up where the groomsmen ran to the bridesmaid and she lifted him up.

Once all the speeches were over, everyone made their way onto the dance floor to get the party rolling. Steven and Nikki provided a photo box for the evening so that we could have everlasting memories of the fun night we had together.

Now married, Nikki became a natural extension of the friendship I had with Steven. I was so blessed and honoured to be a part of their special day and extremely grateful to have both of them, including their family, as a part of my life. It all started with a handshake and turned into a friendship of a lifetime and many more future memories to be made.

Marriage Royale

On Saturday, October 3rd, 2015, was a very special day for the Scott family; it played host to the first marriage within the grandchildren of my family. For those who don't know, wrestling has been a part of my family which you will read more about later in the book. My eldest cousin, Matthew, was locking down his "tag team partner," Ashley, after wrestling/dating each other for four years.

Matthew, whom I also call Macho Man, is just as big a wrestling fan as anyone, so it was only natural for their wedding to have a bit of wrestling flair woven into it. Even though the wedding was predominantly rustic country themed, things like the program and other little details pertained to wrestling and other paraphernlia the couple loved.

The wedding was being held at the Knollwood Golf and Country Club in Ancaster, Ontario. While we were waiting for the ceremony to start, I read through their program that was designed to look like an old wrestling match poster, with "Marriage Royale" in bold letters across the top. I guess you can say we had good seats for the "match" since we were in the front row.

After exchanging vows and officially being married by the "special guest referee" (the officiator), we made our way to the reception area. The interior of the clubhouse was all decorated and cozy. Lots of wood, pumpkins and other fall colours to give an intimate atmosphere. They had a huge homemade dessert table filled with cookies and other treats, including cookies shaped as Hulk Hogan and Macho Man Randy Savage.

Attempting to get the night started, the master of ceremonies and Matthew's best man, Aaron, was having technical difficulties with the microphone. Once Aaron gained control, he did a one, two, three mic test and yelled out the scariest and loudest "Hello!" I've ever heard. My mom's back was to the podium and she jumped right out of her seat, not expecting a thundering voice to ring out. We all had a good laugh at that moment. My cousin Brittany was actually filming me doing something at the time, but she caught my mom's reaction on film so we could relive the moment.

Once the speeches were over, it was the DJ's turn to get the party rocking. Both Matthew and Ashley had a playlist all picked out with their favourite songs and ones that they knew would be a hit. One of Matthew's moments of the night was dancing to one of his favourite movie's theme songs, "Ghostbusters." It was October, near Halloween, and knowing how spontaneous both Matthew and Ashley are, this didn't feel out of place at all.

Since the guests could request songs, I requested "Shout" by the Isley Brothers. This was a special song to Ashley and me because we had danced to this song at my aunt Lorna's wedding the previous year. When our jam came on, Ashley and I both looked at each other and we wheeled ourselves out to the dance floor. Around we went, dancing up a storm. A crowd gathered around us to cheer us on. Everyone loved the moment and came up to tell us how much they enjoyed it.

Matthew and I are cousins, separated in age by five years. As kids, we were pretty close as my dad and his mom were brother and sister. We would play with action figures and video games together and often go on day trips to places like the local wave pool. We drifted apart during the pre-teen/teenage years because of our difference in life stages, but also because of some family dynamics that were happening.

There has been no shortage of drama in the Scott family and Matthew has told me that during those years he felt like an outcast because of how his parents would behave. He felt like doors were closed to him by association and if he were to still talk to certain family members, he would have to deal with being seen as a "traitor" by his own parents. We never held it against him and even he admits how stupid it all was to be standoffish, but when you're a teenager and young adult, you don't always know how to handle those delicate situations. It wasn't until Ashley came into the picture that the relationship with our family was rekindled. She bridged the gap and told us how he felt embarrassed and estranged despite not wanting to, and we organically came back together again after years apart.

Some of my favourite memories of Matthew happened on a trip to Florida in 2003. We were able to connect again after so many years and we bonded over our love of professional wrestling. There was an evening where my dad, Matthew and I were in the outdoor condo pool enjoying the nice weather when a lady in the pool asked us if we were brothers. We looked at each other and scrutinized the woman to see if she was joking, but she wasn't. My dad took it as a compliment and let her off easy by saying we're all related, but realistically my dad was forty-two at the time, Matthew was eighteen (he looked twenty-five with his goatee) and I was thirteen. She was on something because you could clearly see we were all wildly different ages.

The next day, Matthew and I were on the condo balcony with Stirling having lunch overlooking an ocean view. In typical Scott family fashion, we decided to be mischievous by throwing sliced pickles over the railing and into the pool below where people were swimming. We never looked down to see if anything came of it and didn't hear any yelling, but Stirling loved it because it's the type of thing he would have instigated. That's part of our family's sense of humour; we're mischief-makers.

We first met Ashley when she came to my uncle Gordon's annual Celtic Pipe Band Fundraiser in 2010. I was delighted how she was very approachable and friendly. I wasn't even in the building for more than three minutes and we were already chatting away. From that night on, we built a cousin "in-law" relationship. We've shared many laughs and tear-jerking moments together over the years and I'm happy to have her as a part of the family.

Leafs—Sabres Tradition Continues

Ever since my friend Steven and I graduated from Mohawk, one of the traditions we started was going to the Leafs-Sabres game in Buffalo, New York. This particular time in April 2017 was an exciting event for us because it was the first time we got to see the Leafs' young guns Auston Matthews, Mitch Marner and William Nylander play in before our eyes. But we had quite the adventure even before the game started.

We showed our tickets to an arena employee who asked us how in the world we would make it up there. "Where are we sitting?" Steven asked. The employee pointed to the second last row from the very top of the building. It turned out that our seats were in the 300 level and we hadn't noticed. Steven and I looked at each other ready to do this thing. We eventually made it to our seats with the help of Steven's cousin who came along. Settling in our seats, we started laughing at how far up we were. "We're never buying in this section again! We need a beer!"

The Leafs became known for their ability to force a strong offence but outdid themselves when they scored three goals in a span of forty-three seconds in the first five minutes of the first period. After the Leafs started the game strong with a 3-0 lead, one of our fellow Leafs fans, who was sitting behind us literally against the concrete wall, shouted, "Go home, Buffalo!" I turned around and said, "They are home!" Everyone around us erupted with laughter.

After two periods, the Leafs still retained their lead but Buffalo snuck in a goal to make the game 3-1. We decided to get out of our seats to move around and grab another beer when the buzzer went off. We bumped into one of Steven's friends, Tyler, who is a Sabres fan and has season tickets. I loved to tease Tyler for being a Sabres fan. I would ask him why he would buy season tickets if they couldn't win games and tell him his team had the ugliest jerseys. "Ty, you know there's always room for more Leaf fans."

The third period was about to start and even though I abused him, Tyler told us that his section had empty seats we could steal. His section was on the same level, but on the opposite side with a better view.

Toronto dominated from start to finish, outshooting the Sabres 45-22, ending in a 5-2 win. As Steven, Tyler, Steven's cousin and I were waiting for the elevator, there was a guy waiting with us that was likely a Sabres fan, but was wearing a different jersey. I tapped Ty and with a giggle said, "Look Ty, his jersey is much better than yours."

Tyler gave a hopeless expression and said, "You won't lay off on me, will you Kyle?"

I laughed and said, "Nope."

Anna's Not-So-Near-Death Experience

Our D'Agostino Christmas summer gathering has been in full effect for the last few years, its always great to spend quality time with everyone.

My uncle Joe, aunt Janice, cousin Mark and second cousin Daniel love coming down from Ottawa and Kingston, Ontario. They would arrive early on Saturday afternoon to enjoy the day in Uncle Tony and Aunt Susan's pool. Everybody would be in the pool, swimming, floating, playing pool basketball or up on the patio enjoying the sun and sharing conversations until dinner was ready.

On Sunday morning, we're back at the house for breakfast and in the pool for the day. This year, however, several minutes before we were about to come out of the pool, Aunt Anna, who's sometimes afraid of water, had an oh so tragic incident in the pool. She was on an enormous doughnut float relaxing and enjoying the sun. She misjudged her balance when she got off the float and flipped backwards. She went right under and came up in a panic.

My dad, Mark and I were chatting in the deep end when this went down but didn't move an inch. Joe and Tony were up on the patio sitting comfortably on the lounge, looked over, and also did nothing. However, Janice, who was playing basketball with Daniel just inches away from where Anna flipped, quickly reached over to help her regain her balance. In three and a half feet of water, Anna claimed that she almost drowned. We didn't feel like she was in any danger, but she carried on until Janice grabbed her arm to tell her that she's alright and that she got her in time.

"Did you see a bright light, Anna?" my dad teased. She said no and my dad responded, "Then you didn't almost drown!"

My aunt Janice hit my dad and told him to stop it. Anna stayed rooted in her lawn chair for most of the afternoon only to tempt fate in the water again later in the day.

Meeting My Womsis

My best friend James had been seeing a young woman named Sarah for a while. He told me about her one summer's day while sitting on one of our favourite benches near the Chedoke escarpment stairway. Based on what James was saying, I could tell she was the one for my "wombro" and that she would be the person he would marry. James wasn't so sure about it at the time, but I knew because Wombat Junior knows everything.

It took a while for James to bring Sarah around so I could meet her and give my "womproval." After many attempts, we finally met on the first Sunday in February 2018 on a very icy day. Even the weatherman asked everyone to be careful because of the ice. However, we didn't listen. James, Sarah and I went to do a few errands before we stopped at a McDonald's to eat so Sarah and I could get to know each other.

The entire afternoon was filled with stories of James and I growing up including our wombat story, her stories from high school then to favourite TV shows and life in general. I looked at James and said, "Have you told Sarah yet?"

Sarah was intrigued. James gave a smile and asked, "Are you sure? Do you want to do this now?"

Poor Sarah looked a little worried. I wanted to do the honours so I said, "Sarah, I would like to officially crown you as my 'womsis.'"

Sarah's face changed to a huge smile and she said, "I'm totally honoured. I'm happy to meet and get to know one of James's longest, childhood friends who will also become part of my life."

When Sarah went to throw out our garbage, I looked at James and with a straight face said, "Wombro, may I say something to you? I like Sarah!"

Relief poured over his face and he responded, "I'm so happy to hear that, wombro. I value your opinion and wanted there to be a good connection between you two. That's all I could have asked for."

Ms. Kerri "Underwood"

In 2018, my brother Stirling had been seeing someone named Kerri. When the two of them had made their relationship official, my mom and I briefly met her outside as we came home. Kerri got out of her car and walked up to the driveway to introduce herself to my mom. It was extremely respectful of her to do that, and the fact that she went out of her way to introduce herself to me gave me a lot of respect for Kerri. Stirling's previous girlfriend didn't acknowledge me and was disrespectful toward all of my family and friends, so Kerri was a massive upgrade.

At the time, my dad hadn't met Kerri yet, so on a Saturday night in March, we had our first family dinner with Ms. Kerri "Underwood" as I called her. My cousin Matthew joined us as well since he was in town for the day. We all had a wonderful evening getting to know each other. Kerri and I were having great conversations, and once we both realized we loved chocolate and red wine — *we both knew that we wouldn't have a problem getting along.*

In the past few years, Kerri and I have developed a "brother-sister" bond. She is like the little sister I never had. We celebrate, we laugh, we create new adventures, we tease one another, and best of all, we raise our glasses of red wine and salute the chapters of celebration that are in store for our future journey. Kerri is the most approachable, respectful and easygoing young woman you could ever meet and I give her my stamp of approval.

Memories and Celebrations That Will Last a Lifetime

Family Reunites After Forty-Four Years

Our yearly family gathering was started by my uncle Gordon four years ago so we would all be together and celebrate the anniversary of my late grandparents' wedding. In April 2018, our cousins from the States came up for an award that our cousins and their brother Byron received. Since hearing of their trip, Gordon made sure to have the gathering on a weekend when they were in Ontario.

The day before the gathering, we made our way down to Niagara-on-the-Lake to walk along the street that has tons of boutique shops and to enjoy each other's company for an hour until a reservation was ready at Doc Magilligan's Restaurant and Irish Pub. There were about twenty of us all together. I also got to spend time with my brother's new girlfriend, Kerri, and learned more about her. I really liked how she got involved with the family.

Kerri was literally thrown to the wolves with having to meet so many of the family for the first time. Kerri deserves a round of applause for conquering such an intimidating setting.

The next day, we had reservations at Sotiris Greek Restaurant in Burlington for brunch. We rented half of the party room for all thirty family members. This was the first time the majority of the Scott family were together in four-four years. Can you believe it? Uncle Gordon gave a little speech about our family history before we all began to pig out.

After we finished stuffing ourselves, some of us went to visit the gravesite of my grandparents, while others came over to our house to continue the reunion and to watch WrestleMania. Even though the wrestling pay-per-view was a letdown, everyone truly enjoyed the entire weekend together.

My Third Cousin Gets Hitched

The day finally came for my cousin Jeff to marry his love, Erika. I had been looking forward to being a part of their special day for over a year. The wedding was held at a venue called Earth to Table: The Farm on Saturday October 6th, 2018, located not too far from Hamilton. The venue had an open barn with high windows that looked out into rolling hills and farmland.

It was rainy that day, so the wait staff quickly set up chairs inside the building for the ceremony. It ended up being just as beautiful as it would have been outside. Once all the speeches were said, a live band got the party started.

The entire evening was just perfect, from the food, speeches and live music to everyone dancing and enjoying the everlasting memories of Jeffrey and Erika's special day.

Jeff is really special to me and has been an integral part of my life. We've been cousins our entire lives, well, third cousins, but still cousins. I jokingly say that Jeff and I were kept apart growing up for some unknown reason, but we've been told by both sets of parents that we were always busy with sports and other activities while growing up and the Scott family "just didn't want to socialize." It was a joke of course, but everyone did lead busy lives.

After we both graduated high school, we figured to hell with our parents and became close. Thankfully Facebook and MSN Messenger existed because we would use it to communicate on a regular basis while we went to post-secondary. Jeff also attended university in London, Ontario, so I would let him know when I was playing sledge hockey there for a meetup.

The two of us have created a unique bond since befriending each other. We are only two months and two weeks apart in age. Jeff has a charming, joyful and humorous personality, which is similar to my own, but of course, I'm more hilarious. Our journey together has been one filled with laughter, support, understanding and love.

When I met Erika at one of my sledge hockey games in London, I could see the electricity between her and Jeff. I'm happy Jeff found someone to love and love him in return. From that moment on, I knew that we would have a special relationship. Whenever Erika sends me a text asking how I'm doing, it always puts a smile on my face, our conversations are always fun and engaging. Our relationship grew over the years and her personality, love and support made it easy for me to consider her as another cousin. I am extremely grateful to have both of them in my life.

I look forward to creating many more memories together filled with laughter, support, understanding and love.

James's Bachelor Party

On the third weekend of March 2019, eight of us took a trip to Columbus, Ohio, for James's bachelor weekend. We took two vehicles, one going over the Ambassador Bridge (Ontario to Michigan) and another going through the Peace Bridge (Ontario to New York State). My dad and I picked up Tom (James's dad), Dennis (James's cousin) and James at his parent's house at seven in the morning. James's mom, Maureen, asked me to watch over her husband, concerned that he might get a little too tipsy. In the other vehicle were Ben, Ryan, and Marty (Ryan's dad), what a convoy.

After a smooth ride down, we arrived at the hotel in under six and a half hours. The other guys arrived only a few minutes before us, so thankfully nothing happened on the way down to either party. James hates being the centre of attention and since it was his bachelor party, we had the restaurant sing him "Happy Birthday" to make him uncomfortable to start the festivities.

Ben and James were still hungry after just having had lunch, so James, Ben, Ryan and I went to McDonald's. The sidewalk in Columbus was all broken into pieces, lifted a good inch or two off the ground and wasn't accessible, so we had a fun time just walking down the sidewalk on our way to our second lunch.

Whenever I'm with Ben and Ryan, I always feel like I have two personal bodyguards since they've both very tall. Ben is 6'5" while Ryan is 6'8". So you can imagine the four of us rolling into McDonald's with two massive men in front, a guy in a wheelchair and his little chauffeur (James, and I guess I still trust after the incident that happened in grade eight) pushing the chair around. We found a seat, so Ben and James could order the flattest hamburger any of us had ever seen while I enjoyed the simplicity of a strawberry milkshake.

Ben and I have known each other since elementary school, and I've always called him Gentle Ben because he's a gentle giant. I've known Ryan for a shorter amount of time, but we met in high school, while James and

Ben actually played basketball with him when they were kids. Ryan and I have spent quality time together over the years, but for some reason, we just seemed to click with each other during this trip and continue to keep each other on our toes to this day.

Ryan and I were teasing each other in McDonald's, and finally I said with a smirk on my face, "Ryan, do you know what F-U means?"

He looked at me with a smile on his face and, like a smartass, said, "No, Kyle, what does it mean?" That was my way of keeping him in check.

We went back to the hotel afterwards and then up to the room to rest, watch one of the games and chill out. Ryan went to his room for a bit to rest and came right back several minutes later. "Oh, not you again," I said when he came back in. He looked at me like he wanted to throw down. I laughed and said, "You may be tall, but I'm tougher!"

During breakfast the next morning, and I'll just say I haven't seen so much variety in a complimentary breakfast before, we started singing "Happy Birthday" again to James, which everyone else around us joined in on too. It was a nice bright and early embarrassment.

When we arrived at the Nationwide Arena for a basketball game and went through security, a mature security guard said I couldn't go through. My dad asked why. She said that she didn't have the proper equipment to scan me. "Seriously? We have to go back out there, go all the way to the other end and wait in line again?" my dad complained.

She looked at us, thinking. "Yeah, you're right," she said and guided us through to the front of the line where we were supposed to be.

The first game was Iowa against Tennessee. After the first half, Tennessee was leading the game 44-19. Once the second half began, Iowa nearly pulled off another NCAA historic comeback, sending it to overtime to tie at 71 apiece. It was the first overtime game in this year's tournament, but Tennessee managed to beat Iowa 83-77 in overtime.

The second game we saw was Washington against North Carolina. After the first half, UNC was leading 41-33, but they got their stuff together for the second half, pulling together a 13-0 run over five minutes, beating Washington 81-59. As you probably know, I'm not a huge basketball fan, but I respect the game. James has always shown his passion for the game as long I have known him; I remember playing basketball during recess being his "personal defender" along with Ben. However, since my experience attending the March Madness games, I have watched more basketball games than I have had in my whole life. Especially when the Raptors won their first NBA championship title. Even though, in my eyes, hockey is a better sport than basketball (I always tease James about that), I would definitely attend another March Madness game — HECK, an NBA game!

On the way to and from the Nationwide Arena, we took the city bus. It was jammed packed with everyone coming from the game, so we didn't waste this opportunity. We sang ourselves another glorious rendition of "Happy Birthday," which sounded louder than ever because of the bus's confined space. A guy beside me said to the person he was with that, "This is the second time I heard people singing for this guy's birthday."

The area that we were in had a lot of German history. Every building and the surrounding homes were very clean with not a mark on the brick, but the sidewalks were terrible. We walked a block and a few streets over to have dinner at this restaurant called Old Mohawk. We had a great meal, very filling and tasty. We told our waiter that it was James's birthday and ordered him a special drink.

The inside of the building had character: high ceilings, old doors, rustic but cozy. We ate like kings. shorty after, we walked down the street and found a local pub called Wunderbar. The guys got a drink, and we had a few more laughs. Tom got his drink paid for by a lady at the bar, which made him think he "still had it" until the waitress told him that the lady was a sales rep for the beer company and always took care of the tab for anyone drinking one of her drinks.

Back at the hotel, we chilled out again in the lounge and watched the highlight of the day, the March Madness games. My dad was talking to this lady we had seen around for the past two days who asked how we all knew each other. My dad explained that we were here for James's bachelor party. Her reaction was, "Oh, I thought it was his birthday." My dad explained that his groomsmen wanted to embarrass James as much as possible. She laughed and said, "Well, they did a great job. It was the fourth time I heard it," and proceeded to count the four times we actually did sing it. This lady was somehow around every time we broke into song. Was she following us around or was it a coincidence? We will never know.

Kyle N. Scott

The Family Gambling Business

I promised my cousin Samantha that when she turned nineteen, I would take her to a casino for her birthday. Finally, ten long months after her birthday because of her schooling, we set a date and went to Fallsview Casino for dinner, gambling and a show. We all went to the 21 Club Steak and Seafood Restaurant above the casino overlooking the falls and had an incredible dinner before heading to the casino for the moment both Samantha and I were waiting for: playing her first slot machine.

Everybody thinks my dad and I have "tricks" when we play the slots. We really don't. We just put money in and have faith. I brought Samantha to one of my favourite machines and let her play. She won a little bit of money right away and I told her never to play her winnings. She cashed out and went to watch my aunt Susan and my mom play on a machine nearby. I jumped on a machine myself and, of course, after three hits, I won $430. The look on my uncle Tony's face was priceless. Samantha was floored too. "Sam, there are no tricks," I told her. "You put the money in and hit the button. Why go to work when you can do this?" Samantha did pretty well for herself and walked out of there $300 richer.

The show that was playing that evening was called "Midland: A Country Band." Samantha was a little skeptical about the show because she didn't care for country music, but she ended up enjoying the concert and had lots of fun.

"All and all, it was an experience I'll never forget," I remember her telling us. "I will never understand how Kyle and Uncle Colin make all that money, but I can only hope one day I can experience that sort of luck." It was a great start to her gambling career and we promised to take her again in the future.

Wombro and Womsis Get Hitched

Just a few days before my wombro's wedding, James's parents, Tom and Maureen, hosted a rehearsal dinner for the wedding party and associated families. They had a beautiful spread set up in their "Paradise Oasis" of a backyard that faces a beautiful, open green space with a colourful and lush landscape tended by Tom.

As I've mentioned in other stories, Ben, Ryan, Dennis and I were the groomsmen and Tom was the best man. Ryan and I have had a friendly rivalry that we started a few years back, but we really built it up during our bachelor party trip to Ohio. At the rehearsal dinner, I finally got to meet Ryan's fiancée, Alexis. She told me she had heard so many great things about me and how happy she was to finally meet me. I looked over at Ryan after she said that and said, "Oh, so you do love me after all?" Later in the evening, I confessed to Ryan, that I liked Alexis better than him.

"Good, because if you didn't like her more than me, we would have a real problem," he shot back.

During the evening, one of the bridesmaids asked Ryan what I did for a living. "He's a drug dealer," he said laughing. I rolled with it and jokingly said "Perfect!"

James and Sarah said a thank-you speech, followed by Tom welcoming Sarah into the family. As everyone started to clean up and gave their goodbyes, Alexis told me how nice it was to spend the evening with me and that she would see me Friday. I told her that I would look after Ryan for her during the day, but she needed to make sure he was on time. "Don't worry," she said. "I'll have him up early then he's all yours."

Once everyone left, my womsis, Sarah, and I spent quality time together enjoying the beautiful weather. With everything cleaned up, everyone began sharing stories and laughs, including showing Maureen an app called FaceApp, which alters photos to show you what you would look like at different ages. Shortly after, Maureen asked if I had been to or was willing to go to Punta Cana, which I actually was planning to head down to later in October.

"Aren't you afraid of what is happening to Americans who are getting shot or killed over there?" she asked with concern.

"Well, there's only one way to find out!" I jokingly said in return. Everyone had a good laugh and Maureen slapped my arm and told me not to say such things.

James popped up and said, "Well, at least we know what you would have looked like in your old age."

As Ben, Ryan and I were getting ready to leave, Maureen asked what we wanted to drink for breakfast. Ben and Ryan gave their requests before pointing to me. "Alcohol!" I proclaimed.

"Nooooo, Kyle. I meant with your breakfast," she corrected.

I paused for a few seconds and said, "Hmmm, alcohol!"

Everyone laughed. "I love this guy!" Tom proclaimed. Maureen sort of gave in and offered to put Baileys in everyone's coffee.

I looked at her to say, "Maureen, I'll have Baileys... straight up!"

The next morning, two days away from the wedding, I texted Maureen thanking her for a lovely evening.

Friday July 26th, 2019 finally came... the day of the wedding! The guys met at Tom and Maureen's house again and the girls were at a bridesmaids' house. As my dad and I came in, we saw four coolers full of all kinds of alcohol. Tom asked James, "Don't you think you bought a little too much alcohol?"

He said, "Don't worry! There will be less left over than you think and anything left over can be kept or returned."

With James looking as handsome as ever, the photographer finished up their photos of us before we hopped onto the "Magic School Bus." When we arrived, we greeted the guests and showed everyone to their seats.

After a beautiful ceremony and heartfelt speech from the priest, my life-long friend, James, married Sarah, becoming Mr. and Mrs. Wombat. We all ran down the aisle quickly and onto the bus, so we didn't get held up by anyone. As soon as everyone got in, one of the bridesmaids turned on some music and handed out beverages. The song playing had some pretty foul language going on. My dad looked at Tom, who moved his glasses down to the bridge of his nose, and he looked back at him. Without saying a word, they both thought the same thing, "Are you kidding me?" Tom looked around and noted the amount of alcohol that was already flowing and said, "Maybe James was right earlier!" The ride was definitely a long one.

Between the ceremony and reception, we went to the Royal Botanical Gardens, which is the largest botanical garden in Canada, to get pictures of the wedding party, and more importantly, the newlyweds. After a few hours of that, we made our way to the Michelangelo Banquet Centre on the Hamilton mountain. Even though we were running a bit behind schedule, we were able to get there with enough time to enjoy the antipasto bar before the guests were let in.

As all the guests were greeted into the reception hall, the wedding party went to a waiting room for a short break and to discuss the entrances and evening plans. The room itself fit two people comfortably, so imagine what it looked like with the entire wedding party all crammed in there. The DJ knocked on the door, letting the wedding party know that it was "show time." Once the DJ got everyone's attention for us to enter the hall. Ben, Ryan and I said to James, "are you ready for the night of your life?!" The groomsmen made the first entrance, dancing to "Sharp Dressed Man" by ZZ Top accompanied by the beautiful bridesmaids to "Spice Up Your Life" by Spice Girls and James's parents making their way through with their favourite song "Still The One" by the group from the 70's called, Orleans followed by Sarah's mom with "Walking on Sunshine" by Katrina and the Waves. Finally, the bride and groom danced to "September" by Earth, Wind and Fire to begin the night.

Dinner was served while the speeches were underway to provide a little bit of entertainment. I actually had an opportunity to give a speech, which my dad recited for me because of my articulation issues.

My speech was as follows:

> Good evening everyone, my name is Kyle Scott, and I am one of James's lifelong friends. I would personally like to thank everyone here tonight for joining us in celebration of two wonderful people, Sarah and James, as they become husband and wife.
>
> As a long-time friend of James since grade one, I am so proud and honoured to be a part of his special day. From grade one to grade four, our relationship as friends began to tighten. However, the friendship was sealed, specifically, in grade four when we were working on a project for our geography class.
>
> This project created a nickname for the both of us that we still use today. The project itself was about wombats, a creature found in Australia. We spent many moments laughing at such a funny-looking animal and decided to create our own nicknames modelled after them.

Even though I'm six days older than he is, James wanted to be Wombat Senior, which instantly made me Wombat Junior.

As our friendship grew over the years, we had some great school trips that we shared, like when we went to Ottawa, Québec, Toronto Island and many others. One of our many memorable moments was actually in Québec.

As you all might already know, James is a very attentive young man, so James thought he would offer to push me in the wheelchair. I only needed a wheelchair for long distances at that time, but James was excited to help out, and I thought, "Hey great. Time to BOND in Québec." I was enjoying the smooth ride with my new assistant when my driver JAMES decided to spice it up a little. The wind began to flow through my always styled hair; however, every strand of hair on my head began to separate with the speed that I was beginning to experience.

I couldn't hold onto the handles with my hands, so I began to pray for my life, as BOND, JAMES BOND took me for the ride of my life. As the concrete sidewalk began to quickly narrow, seeing the edge coming closer to my Hot Wheels, my beautiful brown eyes began to bulge with the understanding that this could be it. I was going down with the great Double-O-Seven as we crashed in spectacular fashion.

As you can see today, neither of us was any worse for wear after the crash. However, it did leave me lying on the ground and not six feet under it in our rich soil, slightly stained green from the grass, and accompanied by many laughs. But because of that near-death experience, I always request proof of a driver's licence before allowing someone to push me in my wheelchair. See James, you're always teaching me life skills.

I am a sucker for punishment. When we turned twenty-one, we thought, "Let's celebrate big." This might have included revisiting the wheelchair scenario; however, the time had moved on and I already purchased a safety belt.

So, Las Vegas, here we came. We saw things like Bellagio Fountain, Cirque du Soleil Mystère and Kà, Blue Man Group, Louie Anderson, oh yeah, uhhhm, ya, huh, we had a good time! You know what they say, WHAT HAPPENS IN VEGAS, STAYS IN OUR HEARTS... oh, and also IN VEGAS!

James was someone who had many friends in school, but the one thing he would always do is find time out of his social circle to search me out to spend quality time with me, even if it was just to ask "Are you okay, Kyle? Are you having a good time?"

Most of us here tonight obviously share the same emotions and thoughts when it comes to James. He is engaging, always interested in you as a person and your thoughts. He's non-judgmental, always sincere and caring. He is a mentor in many ways; he has compassion for learning, helping others to strive to reach their goals, maximizing their potential. If you could count on one person to have your back, it would be James.

James, I hope you know you can count on me as much as I know I can count on you.

When James started telling me about this young lady named Sarah, I just knew that he had found the special one, and I looked at James and said, "You're going to marry Sarah."

The first time I met Sarah, we spent some quality time getting to know each other, and on that same day, I crowned Sarah as my wombat sister or "womsis" as I call her. She has joined the wombat family that James and I created as kids.

Sarah, you and I know what a great person James is, and we both share a love and respect for him. The fact that we both care for James so much shows that you and I have great taste. You've found your soulmate, your husband, and a lifelong friend, and through

James, I've also gained another great friend in you. I've always been able to count on James, and I know he will never let you down, so take care of each other.

I would like to take this opportunity to raise our glasses for a toast to James and Sarah, to a marriage filled with love and exciting journeys, but most of all to remain open with one another, communicate, love and respect, and oh, it would not hurt to name your firstborn son after me. But if it's a girl, I'm okay with you calling her Kylie.

Love always,

Your Wombro.

With the beautiful and often funny speeches over, the DJ started off with a slow dance and everyone made their way onto the dance floor. All of a sudden, I saw Alexis coming over to me to pull me out with her. Ryan gave me a "Seriously, Kyle?" look and walked away with a smirk on his face.

Ben's girlfriend, Becky, came over to officially introduce herself to me and joined Alexis and I as we were dancing to classics like "Shout," "Hey Jude," "My Girl," and "Stop in The Name of Love." Ryan and Ben both shook their heads while standing on the sidelines before eventually joining us, along with Sarah and James.

Alexis and I started a conga line that got literally everyone out of their seats. Alexis and I made a super long line, which many claimed was the best conga line ever created because it got so many people involved. When the line first started to materialize, the DJ looked over at us and thought, "Oh yeah! This is happening!"

Then there was Tom's eighty-year-old aunt, standing maybe five foot two, 110 pounds, who made our night. While I was dancing with James's sister Melanie, her great-aunt asked if she could dance with me. I wasn't going to turn her down and boy, could she rock the dance floor. She danced with every muscle in her body and took me for a ride that reminded me of a trip I once had in Florida where I rode the Magic Teacups at Disney. She had me spinning in all directions, and just enough to keep me from throwing up.

Memories and Celebrations That Will Last a Lifetime

Melanie made several attempts to help pry me from granny's rockin' grip as she saw that I had had enough of that ride. Melanie was gracious about it, thanking her great-aunt and briskly wheeling me away. I ended up at one of the tables my parents were sitting at only for a few seconds because the rockin' granny swept me back onto the dance floor.

That night, she danced the night away, putting a lot of young ones to shame. She knew every word to every song. Even newer ones like "The Git Up" by Blanco Brown. "The only time I will stop moving is when I'm dead!" Yes, she said those very words to us.

Everyone in attendance was compatible, respectful, classy and sincere to each other. They enjoyed themselves and the dance floor was filled right until the end, which is what I love to see at these events. I loved this wedding and loved being a part of my best friend's special day. All I have left to say is, "Wombats forever!"

Growing up with Wombat Senior has been truly memorable and life-changing since the very first day we met in elementary school. You rarely stay friends with someone from such a young age, and I'm truly blessed to have our remarkable "womship" (friendship) for twenty-four years and counting.

We both created a special bond unlike any other that will last forever, no matter who goes first (I always remind him that "I'm going first" because I don't want to cry at his funeral). We have been through many ups and downs together throughout the years and have always been there for one another.

When James asked me to be one of his groomsmen and stand beside him while he married the love of his life, not only was I honoured, but it made me feel incredibly special to him. Sarah became a natural part of our already existing womship too, so now we're a "womthree."

The memories that we shared over the years are unforgettable. Memories of the bachelorette party — I mean bachelor party weekend — right up to the wedding day will stay with me forever.

I look forward to creating new cherished memories with the two of them in the years to come. Wombats forever!

Chapter 11: Trips and Adventures

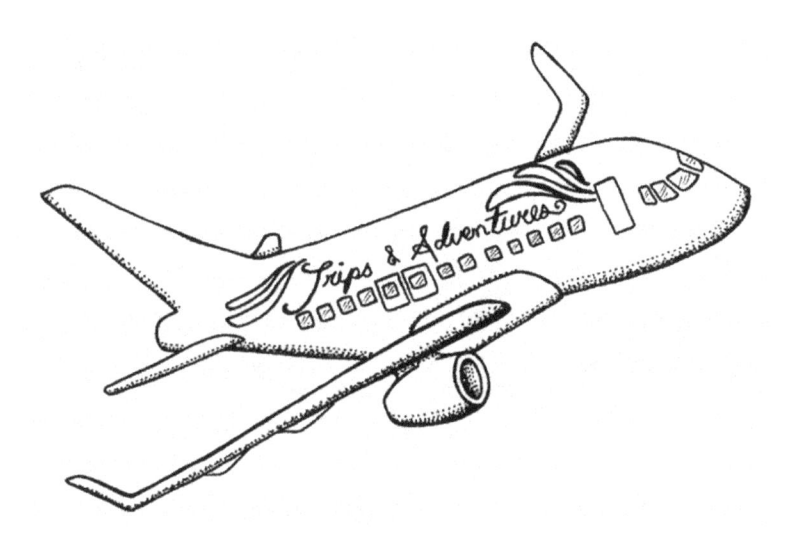

My Hockey Heroes

My uncle Tony bought two tickets for my dad and me to see the Toronto Maple Leafs take on the New York Islanders back on March 28th, 1998, at what used to be the Maple Leaf Gardens. This was a thank-you gift for being the ring bearer at his wedding and it happened to be my first live hockey game. My dad called the public relations office ahead of time and told them how much passion I had for the game of hockey.

Seated on level 300, my dad and I walked up to the first set of stairs. My dad gave our tickets to one of the arena assistants who looked at them and, with an unexpected attitude, said, "Are you kidding me?" My dad asked him what the issue was and the assistant snorted, "You guys are all the way up there? I'm going to have to take the wheelchair and put it away." My dad was obviously annoyed at this point, but responded with, "You do what you have to do, sir." Our seats didn't have complete wheelchair access to them, so we had to walk a part of the way up to them while the assistant stored the chair in a locked room.

Once we got up to our seats, which were pretty high up and steep, we ended up sitting with fans from out west who were very nice and chatty throughout the game. My dad told them how much I loved hockey and the Leafs. He even told them about his call to the PR office, who would eventually come and get us for something special. They absolutely didn't believe my dad in the slightest. With five minutes left in the third period, one of the PR employees, whom I will refer to as "PR guy" from now on, came and pointed to us from a platform, knowing exactly where we were sitting. The out-of-town fans couldn't believe it as we left our seats.

The game was tied at three apiece by this point, so the tension was pretty high as we made our way down to the ice after we got my wheelchair back. The assistant who had the key to the locked room was nowhere to be found, so the PR guy had to call him repeatedly to open the room. Finally back in my chair minutes later, the PR guy explained where we were going and brought us right to where the players came off the ice when the game ended. I remember him saying something along the lines of, "This is where the Leafs will come off the ice. Don't go up to them. Let them come to you. Also, if they lose, you may see some sticks flying around and if they win, well that's a good thing!"

The game went into overtime and the Leafs beat the Islanders 4-3. I watched the entire Leafs roster come off the ice teeming with excitement and amped up from the overtime win. The Leafs captain at the time, Mats Sundin, came up to introduce himself, shook my hand and said, "Nice to meet you, Kyle! Did you enjoy the game tonight?" Whoa, did that really happen? Thankfully, I got a great picture with him to prove it.

It didn't stop there because a few minutes later Wendel Clark introduced himself too and said, "I want you to have this stick I cracked tonight!"

Wendel had signed the stick before giving it to me and it's still on display in my room to this day.

Once the Leafs went into their dressing room, the head coach back then, Mike Murphy, came out of his office to speak to me. He shook my hand and looked at my homemade flag hat, which looked more like a flag twisted into a dunce cap, to be honest. "Nice hat, Kyle!" Mike laughed. "I actually brought you a new Maple Leafs hat right here, so get rid of this thing you have on."

I was completely thrilled to meet so many of my hockey heroes. The PR guy said, "Okay guys, let's go in!" My dad and I both looked at him, confused, and asked, "Uh, where too?" He smirked and said, "Into the Leafs dressing room!"

When we arrived in the locker room, all the players knew me by name and shook my hand. I had the privilege of meeting players like Tie Domi, Steve Sullivan, Sergei Berezin, Danny Markov, Alyn McCauley, Mike Johnson, Fredrik Modin, Derek King and Glenn Healy. The only player I didn't have the chance to meet was Félix Potvin, whom I pretended to be when I played goalie during floor hockey, Potvin was actually in the tub at the time, but we still managed to get his autograph.

Each time a player came up to shake my hand and sign their autograph, my dad kept turning my jersey to keep the signatures balanced out. We were both amazed and grateful for such a once-in-a-lifetime opportunity to meet the entire Toronto Maple Leafs team.

I'm really appreciative of what the PR guy did for us that day. My dad even said that he went above and beyond his expectations. This was such a wonderful experience that I will never forget.

Florida Brings Out the Best in Grandparents

Ever since I was fourteen months old, my family and I would go to Florida for vacation. We would always visit my uncle George and aunt Jean who lived down there (Indian Rocks Beach) forty-five minutes from Tampa. In the summer of '99, my nonna came along with us and we decided to drive down.

We are talking about a road trip that would rival Clark Griswold. Keep in mind, Hamilton, Ontario, to Florida is 2,268 km, or twenty-plus hours of driving. For our family, it is usually three days of reasonable driving. I have no idea how some people can go straight through without stopping overnight to sleep!

My brother Stirling was three and a half years old at the time and was a very active kid! Stirling wanted everything and kept bugging and bugging and bugging my dad to pull over. He was most likely tired and cranky from the long ride. We stopped on the side of Interstate 75 and my dad went to the opposite side of the van to talk to Stirling. Nonna was sitting in the seat closest to the sliding door and could see my dad was holding something in his hand; a sandal. The door would open slightly and then immediately shut again. Again, it would open and then shut. My dad couldn't see what Nonna was doing and didn't have a clue.

Nonna thought for sure that my dad was going to hit Stirling with the sandal, so she was doing what she had to as a grandmother to protect her grandson. I guess if you see someone with a sandal in hand, and the other is on a foot, you would think something was about to go down. My nonna defused the situation that day by stepping in. I didn't say it out loud, but I wanted to say, "Way to go, Nonna," even if Stirling was getting on everyone's nerves.

One afternoon, my family and I had decided to order pizza for lunch. There was a pizza place down from our condo on Gulf Boulevard, so we had easy access. My dad, Nonna, and I walked to get the pizza on what seemed to be a normal, sunny day. If you've never been to Florida, just know that weather can stir up and down out of nowhere without warning.

With pizza in hand, making our way back to the condo, a massive black cloud was forming above our condo. It was like a scene from a movie. We picked up the pace and moved as fast as we could. We were maybe halfway home when Nonna handed us the pizza box and, in broken English, said, "Here, go without me. Run, leave me behind!"

Finally, we made it to the condo parking lot just as the sky dumped everything it had on us. Massive puddles began to form everywhere. Since I was in my wheelchair, my dad soldiered through the water, literally parting it like the Red Sea, but to my nonna, it looked like we had lost control and were going to crash. She sprang into action and started running to save me. When she got close, she saw that we weren't out of control, but were laughing and having a good time. She actually laughed so hard at the situation that she peed her pants.

Every day, my dad, Stirling and I would be in the pool from 9:00 a.m. to 5:00 p.m. It was like that Dolly Parton song, swimming nine to five. Sometimes after dinner, depending on what went on, my dad wanted me to practise holding my breath underwater to help with my lung capacity. Once I was able to hold my breath for twenty seconds or more, I was able to take on the next step, venturing into the deep end. My dad would hoist me up onto his back with my arms wrapped around him or place me in front of him holding my waist as we went down to the bottom of the pool. Yes, eight feet under to the bottom of the pool. I remember the feeling of being underwater as being so peaceful and relaxing. I could just float and not worry about how my body normally felt.

My dad's parents were also down in Florida vacationing at the same time. They actually flew down and then drove back home with us when we left. Obviously, the van was a full house with my dad and grandpa in the front, Grandma and I in the middle, and Nonna, Stirling (who was in a car seat) and my mom in the back with all our luggage and a wheelchair. It was completely rammed in there with no stops along the way. My grandfather made us drive twenty-four hours straight because he didn't want to waste time.

At one point, the air conditioner made my grandfather too cold so he decided to take a beach towel and wrap it around his head. People who drove past would stare at him, not expecting to see someone wrapped in a towel. Grandpa asked why everyone looked so shocked and my dad told him he looked like E.T. hiding like in the movie. My grandpa turned his head to peer through a little gap he made and said, "What? I'm cold." Needless to say, this experience never happened again and we were thankful to be out of that car the second we got home.

Everyone felt like a day-old pretzel by the end of it, all seven of us crammed in there surrounded by luggage for twenty-four hours straight. It was an experience that never happened again, to be sure.

Kyle N. Scott

Dominican, Here We Come!

With high school behind me and the 2007 summer season beginning to heat up, my dad wanted to take us on a family vacation of my choosing. I wanted to try something different from the usual trip to Florida that we would normally take. My brother Stirling wasn't too happy when he found out we were going somewhere else. He couldn't believe that we would want to go to an all-inclusive resort instead of staying with our great uncle George and aunt Jean. I remember him saying something like, "Oh great! You picked all the food you can eat and drink over the family." My dad responded sarcastically with, "Yep and you will see that you will love this just as much!"

Fast forward a few weeks and we're boarding a plane to Punta Cana in the Dominican Republic. As we're getting ready for takeoff, a flight attendant knelt down beside our seats to discuss "an emergency matter" with us. She basically wanted to know what the plane staff was required to do to help me in case of an emergency. My dad and I looked at each other with the same expression. "Well, just throw my son out the door," my dad said with a straight face. The flight attendant nearly fell backwards in shock as she wasn't expecting such an answer. My family always goes for the most shocking answer just to see what kind of reaction we get out of people. Of course, we had to show her we were joking even though I was prepared to skydive into the Atlantic Ocean.

The moment we stepped off the plane, the humidity and raw heat slapped us right in the face; something we really weren't expecting. This was our first trip to an all-inclusive resort, so none of us knew exactly what to expect as we pulled up to the Grand Oasis Resort that evening. The resort looked welcoming and beautiful all lit up at night.

The next morning, my dad and I hustled to the beach for the first time. All I could say is that we were in paradise and the view of the beach was breathtaking. My dad rolled me to the beachfront and proceeded to push the wheelchair through the sand. A big mistake because the wheelchair just sank in, bringing us to a halt. While I was marooned in my wheelchair, I took a good look at how beautiful the Caribbean ocean was. I leaned a little too far to the left and flipped out of my chair into the sand. Both my dad and I laughed, trying to get me back up and out of the sand. The entire left side of my body was covered with sand and with everyone watching (looked like a crime scene from CSI). I'm sure they were wondering why we brought a wheelchair in the first place. Neither my dad nor I are physicists and were too enamoured with the landscape to even pay attention to where we were actually walking. So, if it wasn't obvious already, no wheelchairs on sandy beaches if you're reading this.

Even Stirling warmed up to the resort after two days. For the first day or so, you could tell he really didn't want to like the place and would walk around with such an attitude. On that third day, he came up to a table we were at, threw his feet up on it while eating a piece of fruit, and said, "Anytime you want to come here, I'm in!"

My dad and I found out early on in the trip that people who often went to resorts went for a good time and couldn't care less how they were perceived. There was a day where my dad and I went to the adult-only pool hoping to find a quiet place to chill out. We met a young couple in the pool and struck up a conversation with them. I guess the girl felt comfortable because she asked us if we were brothers at one point. My dad jokingly played it off. "I think you might have a vision problem. You may have cataracts, but you look too young for that. Oh, maybe you're drunk!" However, she insisted that we were brothers despite being over twenty years apart. My dad and I don't have much in common appearance-wise. I took after my mom's Italian side, so I look a lot like my mom just with more facial hair than her.

The girls who worked at the resort loved me and would touch the gorgeous, curly hair I had at the time — I used to get perms. Yeah, yeah, I know. When live music rang out throughout the resort, the girls would come over to dance with me. Of course, they would always give kisses and wanted them in return as well. There was one instance where I was laying flat on a lawn chair suntanning and one of the girls took it upon herself to get on top of me claiming to want to have my babies. I looked at my dad and said, "Uh, Grandpa?"

We loved our first all-inclusive experience. The landscape was serene and inviting; the resort welcoming and full of life. It was something we had never experienced up until that point and we've been back quite a several times since then.

Kyle N. Scott

Las Vegas, Here We Come!

With so many things to celebrate in 2010, we decided to plan a trip to Las Vegas. Both James and I were celebrating our twenty-first birthdays, my uncle Gordon was turning fifty and my dad, well, he was just a tag-along guy.

A few weeks before our big trip, I was visiting James. His mom, Maureen, was very paranoid and nervous about her innocent son heading down to Las Vegas with my family. Maureen knew the Scott family for our enthusiastic and captivating senses of humour, but friends of friends were jokingly filling her in on what we were "really going there for," which was the girls. Maureen thought she would have to kiss her son's innocence goodbye.

She brought this up, imploring my dad not to lead her son down the path of sinful delight. My dad assured her that James would be treated as his own son and wouldn't have to worry. That calmed her nerves enough to still let James board the plane with us.

We drove early Thursday morning to the Buffalo Airport in New York to make our flight to Las Vegas. We arrived around 10:30 a.m. While in a cab (and remember, it's our first time in Vegas), we were amazed by the grandeur and spectacle of the place. Our heads were on a swivel, trying to soak everything in. James asked the cabbie how cold it could get out there. The cabbie responded with 13 degrees Celsius in the winter, but over 33 during the day, which is nothing compared to Canadian weather.

We arrived at our home base for the next week, the Flamingo hotel. After unpacking and having some lunch, we hit the strip. At the time, my dad was dealing with painful sciatica in his legs. If you've never been to Vegas, just know that all you do is walk and the buildings aren't as close together as they appear to be. You can't even cross the road. Instead, you have to take elevators, escalators, bridges, and stairs to get across. With all that said, my wheelchair really came in handy as it ended up doubling as a walker for my dad, which helped save him from constant, excruciating sciatic pain.

As we entered the Luxor hotel, we toured the Titanic exhibit that had everything that was found after the historical ship plunged into the depths of the ocean. There was one big piece of the ship that I found fascinating and was kind of in shock to be sitting in front of. Like most museum pieces, there was a sign reading not to touch the display. "Mr. Innocence" James leaned over us and devilishly whispered, "I touched the big piece!"

My dad and I both turned around to say, "You did what? James!" What a scandalous thing to do! As we were almost at the end of the exhibit, there was an original perfume bottle in one of the glass stands that actually had little holes in it to let us smell it. My dad went in for a sniff but had to put his hands on the edge to take the pressure off his legs. Woop, woop! My dad accidentally triggered an alarm. A sea of eyes turned to stare at my dad as if he were trying to break in to steal the perfume. My dad threw his arms up in the air to show he didn't do anything, plus they had cameras everywhere to confirm nothing was going on.

After nearly being arrested for robbery, we hit the other side of the strip to see the different casinos and activities that were happening. I enjoyed the architecture of the buildings, being a designer myself. We watched the Bellagio water show, which was amazing because I found it to be technically fascinating. Caesars Palace was very beautiful with its rows upon rows of torchiere lamps. When we found a pool area called "The Garden of the Gods," we legitimately felt like we were in Heaven among the pure white Roman statues and columns. "If this is what Heaven is like, I'm in!" my dad exclaimed, standing in awe.

Every night, we saw a different show like Mystère by Cirque du Soleil at Treasure Island and the Louie Anderson show at The Excalibur. While standing in line before the show, Louie came out, commenting on how full the house was. He saw me behind everyone and came right over, shook my hand, and thanked me for coming, which was nice of him.

Right after the Louie show, we rushed to get a taxi to head over to the MGM Grand to see Cirque du Soleil's Kà performance. The show was magnificent and the stage itself was working on hydraulics. The performers worked on a stage platform that would go vertical, obviously putting them at risk of falling. I've never seen such physical talent and dedication to art.

Remember earlier when I mentioned James asking the temperature? Well, the next morning, ironically, we stepped outside after having breakfast at the buffet. The temperature was 13 degrees! Can you believe it?

In Vegas? Canadians can experience weather warmer than 13 degrees in April, although we have also seen snow in May!

We started the day off with a taxi ride to Fremont Street to experience what's called Old Las Vegas. We were in one of the stores and James wanted to buy me a t-shirt. He held up a shirt to show my dad, who read it out loud as "Want a good ass licking?"

James was taken a bit aback, swung the shirt around and went, "No, no. It says, 'Want a good ass-kicking?'" He didn't end up buying me that shirt because he said he wouldn't be able to get that graphic image out of his head. However, he did buy me another, much tamer shirt as a gift. I told you how innocent he is.

Shorty after, we went to the Golden Nugget Hotel and Casino to wait for another taxi, while my dad went to a restroom. Not even minutes later, my dad came out holding a piece of paper for us to read. As he came closer, you could clearly see it read $800. "What? Where? How?" For the second time that day, James was taken aback.

"Oh, you know! Money will never change me!" said my dad in response. His tune changed once the taxi rolled up. "I don't want to ride in this. It's old and rusted!"

We took the rust bucket to the Aria hotel for dinner. The receptionist asked for my dad's credit card to pay for the food and called him by his first name, Colin. "Oh no, it's Sir Scott. I just came into a lot of money today." The cashier laughed and called him Colin again to which my dad, again, corrected her. James just stood there shaking his head and asked if this was going to go on for the rest of the day.

In the evening, my uncle Gordon wanted to see Donny and Marie Osmond in our hotel. Dad, James, and I opted to see the Blue Man Group instead at the Venetian hotel. After an awesome show, we returned to Gordon's room to find him lying on the bed watching TV with $110 worth of one-dollar bills stacked on his end table. We thought he had won thousands of dollars and James was once again confused about how the Scott family manages to win money. Before any of us started laughing, my dad threw the money on the bed and started swimming in it like Scrooge McDuck.

It didn't matter what time of day it was, you could find and see everything you wanted on the Vegas strip. We often saw groups of people handing out business cards for escort services that people could dabble in if that was their pleasure. "Mr. Innocence" James decided to collect as many as he could throughout the day as if it were his part-time job... only handing them back out to the people walking on the strip of Las Vegas.

Five days later, we were officially spent and felt like we had experienced everything we could from weather to entertainment, even winning a couple of bucks here and there. Aboard the plane and nearly home, the plane crew began collecting garbage. One of the flight attendants said something to my dad. Curious, we leaned over to ask what she said. "She said you guys are keen bastards." Neither one of us knew what that even meant.

When she came back around again, my dad caught her attention and asked her why she called us such a thing. "What? I didn't say that! I said you guys are clean passengers." My dad played it off by saying his ears were blocked.

Looking back, the entire trip was the most exciting twenty-first birthday celebration anyone could experience. I am glad that I got to experience this adventure with my lifelong friend James and it was an honour to celebrate my uncle Gordon's fiftieth birthday too.

That Man is a Rapist

My aunt Janice threw her husband (my uncle Joe) a surprise sixtieth birthday party in late October 2010. She set it up to take place at the Landings Golf Course in Kingston, Ontario, after they had played a round of golf. When we arrived, Joe was just putting his clubs away in the car. My dad rolled down the window and asked him for directions. Joe turned around with shock to see us.

The birthday also served as a way for all of our family's older generation to meet the younger part of the family. My cousin Mark became a father to his son Daniel a month earlier and had not yet met much of the family. This was my Nonna's first "Pronipote" (great-grandson), finally making her a Bisnonna (great-grandmother).

We were a few hours early and decided to check into the hotel. On our way there, my aunt Anna had to stop at Shoppers Drug Mart to get a birthday card and a few other things. As Anna got out of the van, my dad told her we would wait for her. When Anna went in, my dad moved the van to a parking spot on the opposite side of the entrance. When Anna came out, she stopped dead in her tracks and looked around frantically. You could see the panic and confusion on her face. We had a good laugh and called her over so we could hit the road again.

At the hotel, Anna noticed a door wide open with a man working on his laptop in the far back. We don't always know if Anna is joking or not on the best of times, but she turned around and whispered, "That man knows I'm alone and he's going to come in and rape me."

My dad looked at her and said, "Yeah, Anna. He's been waiting for you all day." I went into our room while my dad walked Anna to hers as a "ruse" to make sure the alleged rapist didn't think she was alone.

You may remember that I previously mentioned that it's super easy to play a prank on Anna and my dad never misses an opportunity. When she came over to our room to hang out, my dad snuck out to Anna's under the guise of taking something to her room for her. In her room, he created a body out of the pillows and threw the sheets back over it to give the appearance that someone was under them. When Anna eventually left our room, my dad counted down three, two, and... one before we heard Anna screaming and banging on her door to get out.

She came running back to our room to say, "Can someone sleep with me tonight?"

I thought "Seriously?" We looked at each other and both Stirling and I told her absolutely not. My dad opted out too, which forced my mom, who had nothing to do with any of it, to take on the responsibility.

Hitting the Strip

One Saturday in May 2012, my high school buddies wanted to celebrate everyone's birthdays at a strip club. I brought my cousin Jeff along for the sights and smells. We had lots of fun catching up with each other since we all led busy lives. After a few girls danced for us, I decided to have one final dance. When the girl approached, I wasn't really into her because she gave off this bad vibe. She was doing her thing but started mouthing off to my friends over how disrespectful it was to bring me a place like this when I didn't know what was happening. Talk about assumptions. I looked over at everyone who was giving me "wacko" signs and to end the dance ASAP. Jeff gave me money which I promptly handed to her while telling her to get off of me. She took it, huffed and left, but a scene had already been created, which other patrons took notice of.

At first, my cousin Jeff felt embarrassed over what the dancer was trying to say. She was making a scene and directing her comments to everyone in the room but me. Most of my friends felt like maybe they did do something wrong, which I quickly dispelled, but we figured out that it wasn't our problem at all; it was hers. She must not have realized what it meant to have a physical disability and how it didn't necessarily mean you were unaware of what was happening. If she had tried to communicate with me, she would have seen that appearances can be deceiving.

Life Is Full of Surprises

Before taking a trip to Punta Cana, we celebrated my mom's sixtieth properly by throwing her a surprise party with nearly everyone she knew. We rented a private room at one of my family's favourite restaurants, Sotiris Greek restaurant.

We began planning it as far back as April of that year, so we were worried about her finding out. However, my aunt Theressa came up with a brilliant idea to convince her that we were going to a '50s/'60s dance at a Holiday Inn nearby that we would check out after dinner at Sotiris.

The staff at Sotiris knows us well from being guests for so many years. Toni, the waitress who served us pretty much each time we ate there, was our waitress supervisor for the party. As usual, Toni greeted us at the door and played along with the ruse. She directed us to the private room and my mom was like, "Why are we going in here?" She opened the doors and, "SURPRISE!"

My mom was stunned and overwhelmed. She sort of stepped back a little as if she were blown back by the surprise. Once it sunk in that the surprise was for her, she turned to us like she wanted to murder us for duping her. "We don't have time for that," my dad jokingly said. "These people want you to come in!"

Everyone there was family and friends that we socialized with throughout my mom's life. It was a wonderful evening and everyone truly enjoyed themselves.

The parents of a grade school classmate of mine named Rick and Silvana (not to be confused with my mom who shares the same name) became really good friends with my parents over the years and wanted to go away with us on vacation in 2016 shortly after the sixtieth birthday party. My dad has an open invitation when it comes to travelling and tells everyone they're welcome to come along.

We went down in July and stayed at Chic Punta Cana by Royalton in the Dominican Republic. The resort is for adults only and it marked the first time we had ever been to that type of resort. On our first full day at the resort, we met a friendly Canadian couple, Brad and Nancy from Aurora, Ontario, after we had breakfast.

We had multiple drinks together, danced, and engaged in many conversations including just how small the world seems at times when you meet someone who lives only an hour or so away. The couple knew folks who lived up the street from us and even stranger still, Silvana and Rick knew those people personally. It really is amazing how small the world is when you are on vacation and you both know of someone from the same hometown.

As you know by now, I love being in the water and when I am on vacation, I am in the water pretty much all day long, except for when we are eating or participating in resort-hosted events. Silvana is a very hyper person. After we finished our lunch one day and went back to our pool area, my dad and I planned a prank for her.

My dad would usually bring me right up to the edge of the pool in the wheelchair and I would jump in. People would think I fell out of my chair and get all panicked. My dad brought me up to the edge like usual and knowing that Silvana fears the water due to a traumatic experience, he called her over to "help" me get in. My dad instructed her to get closer to behind the back of my knees. Silvana ran so quickly, got the chair, and put the seat right under my bottom. I think she thought I needed to sit down, however, she was grossly mistake. We were setting up to think she pushed me into the water with the wheelchair, and mission was accomplished, in I went. I stayed underwater for about thirty seconds to make it look like I was drowning. Above water, Silvana was screaming bloody murder. A random resort guest walked by and asked if we needed help, but my dad let him know we were playing a joke. It took her about half an hour to calm down and get her heart rate back to normal, but it was definitely worth it.

On July 13th, we celebrated my mom's sixtieth birthday by having breakfast at the Ocean Side restaurant on site at the resort. Brad and Nancy came up and sang her "Happy Birthday." Later in the afternoon, Brad came up to me and said, "I really loved watching you actually swimming and doing lengths. Some people can't swim or are afraid of water, so seeing you do what you do with a smile brings my wife and me joy."

There was a very entertaining group of twelve from Nashville who were partying all the time and the younger generation couldn't keep up with them. We were celebrating my mom's sixtieth at the resort's Hunter's Steakhouse and the group had just arrived as we were finishing up our dessert. As I was going by their table, I said, "Hey guys, I just want all of you to know that tonight's dinner is on me!"

They all said, "We really appreciate it, Kyle!"

The very next night, we were having dinner at the Italian restaurant called Vespa and the group from Nashville was already there and just finishing up. As they were leaving, they walked by to return the gesture from the night before. "Hey, our Canadian friends! Just letting all of you know that dinner is on us. Enjoy!" Oh wait, it's all-inclusive.

During our stay, my brother Stirling and I kept getting asked if we were twins. Stirling would visit the resort spa and gym, which required you to sign in. My dad and I went to the spa portion one mid-afternoon for some peace and quiet before having dinner while Stirling was also in the area. As we came in and about to sign in, one of the staff members looked at me and said, "You've signed in already."

My dad laughed and said, "Hmm, that would be his brother." She asked if we were twins like so many others had on this trip. "No, ma'am. Brothers!" my dad corrected.

My dad and I love going to casinos, and we often end up winning money. One of the dealers at the resort casino kept looking at me. She finally mustered up the courage and told me I was good looking and had a wonderful smile. My dad proceeded to pimp me out, offering me the introductory rate of five bucks. She claimed to have no money, so my dad said, "We'll come tomorrow night and I'll offer you a half-off deal until midnight." We had a good laugh about it, but she definitely was pretty.

Before the trip ended, Brad and I exchanged email addresses to keep in touch. A few weeks after we both returned, I mentioned to Brad that my cousin and I were going to a Toronto Blue Jays game. Little did we know, Brad was going to the same game too. We met up and had a beer together, pretending we were still in the Caribbean. Brad got to meet my cousin Jeff and a few weeks later, Brad showed a picture of all of us to this guy he knew who turned around and said, "That's Jeffrey! I went to university with him." It's incredible how connected we are sometimes. You just never know what life brings when you meet people on your vacation.

Lost in Vegas

During the second week of August in 2016, we went back to Las Vegas. It would be my third time since 2010. This time we stayed at Bally's Hotel, which is situated right in the centre of all the action. It was a scorching 41 degrees Celsius while we were there and it only dropped down to about 28 degrees Celsius by nighttime.

Even though we had been down twice, we finally got to see one of the must-see shows in Vegas called "O" by Cirque du Soleil. It's a water-themed stage production that is inspired by the "infinity and elegance of water's pure form." It was one of the most spectacular and breathtaking show I have ever seen. After the show, we were waiting at the crosswalk for the light to change. There was a stampede of people crossing from both sides, at least 150 people. The lady beside us had a look of panic on her face. I remember my dad saying, "It's like the West Side Story. East meets west!"

As we were on our way to Mandalay Bay to see the "Michael Jackson: One" Cirque du Soleil show, we had quite an adventure getting there. We walked from our hotel, Bally's, to the Aria hotel, which took just under twenty-five minutes. We needed to take an elevator at the Dolce and Gabbana building to cross a bridge that would take us to another elevator to go down, but we noticed that the second elevator was out of service. There was no other way to get down to the main strip from the pedestrian bridge unless we went all the way back to the previous bridge several blocks back. My dad turned around and said, "There's no way I'm walking all the way back to crossover and walk back here!" I didn't blame him because it would have taken us another fifteen minutes to get back to the same spot.

We walked back to Dolce and Gabbana to search for an elevator to take us down. Once we finally found our way to the main strip, we thought we would pass through by crossing the street around the corner on West Aria Place. Once we crossed over, we were immediately met by a wall of rod iron fencing and flower beds made of concrete. Apparently, this helps keep people coming in from off the main strip. Gold stars to whoever came up with that idea. We walked through the underground parking area of the Aria Express Park MGM Station and kept walking, hoping we could find a route back to the main strip. As we exited the underground parking, we still didn't succeed. Desperate, Dad said, "Let's try this way," which landed us on Las Vegas Boulevard. Here we were walking on the road as vehicles buzzed by, probably thinking, "What the hell are people doing on the road?" I'm sure security loved watching a guy in a wheelchair being pushed around Las Vegas Boulevard hoping not to get caught, arrested, or run down.

We finally found our way back to Park Avenue, landing at the intersection of Park and Las Vegas Boulevard. At the corner, there was a place called the Shake Shack. "We definitely need a cold shake after that adventure," my dad said. We continued making our way to Mandalay Bay to grab tickets for the Michael Jackson show. The show ended up being amazing. The entire thing was packed with "wow" moments from beginning to end. It was energizing, action-packed and a visual phenomenon, and who doesn't love Jackson's music?

I have been asked by lots of people if I ever get bored with Vegas. My answer: *never!* Las Vegas is an internationally renowned major resort city, known primarily for its gambling, shopping, fine dining, entertainment, architecture, and nightlife, and is now home to two professional sports teams, the Golden Knights and the Raiders.

So it goes without saying that each time you go there, it's always a new experience. You never run out of things to do and I bet you will check out a hockey game and maybe a football game the next time you go there; I know I will.

Remember one important thing, "What happens in Vegas, stays in Vegas!"

A Wombro Weekend

James and I wanted to spend some quality time together ever since he asked me to be a groomsman. I remember him asking me when we were out to dinner and I initially said "no" just to be a jerk.

"Classic Kyle," James said at the time. "Being a big prick when I'm trying to be serious and thoughtful." Anyway, we went to Niagara Falls for our wombro weekend.

We arrived at the hotel and relaxed for what felt like two seconds then made our way to the falls. Murray Street is pretty steep and I'm sure there have been more than a few people who've nearly killed themselves walking up and down it. I warned James to enjoy rolling me down it because coming back will be a good workout. When we hit the bottom, I jokingly mentioned how exhausting it was coming down. "I think I need a nice, cold drink and a little bite to eat."

James gave me a look like, "Are you frigging kidding me? I did all the work!"

We went and ate before walking around the scenic falls area. James wanted to know where I wanted to go, so I told him we could jump into the falls. We decided to take the Hornblower Cruise. We put on ponchos and made our way to the front of the boat. The power of the waterfall was intense with so much water endlessly pouring down around us. We were soaked from head to toe rather quickly, barely managing to get a photo without getting the camera all wet.

Soaked to the bone, we both decided to do zip-lining over the falls next to dry off. They had to get someone to hook me up and make sure I was properly secured. Out of all the workers, this young and beautiful blonde woman around my age came over to hook me up. I looked over at James, who knew exactly what I was thinking, with a huge smile on my face.

What a spectacular ride and amazing feeling. I flew 2,200 feet and clocked over seventy kilometres per hour across a breathtaking and exhilarating view of the American and Canadian Horseshoe Falls.

After we got a ride back up to the top, James asked, "Seriously, how do you do it?" which was in reference to ladies. I laughed and said, "Well, sometimes it's good to have a disability." We went to the Fallsview Casino next by walking up and through Clifton Hill. We stopped at the Grand Buffet in the casino to eat yet again and boy were we hungry. I spent some free play coupons immediately after and managed to cash out at just under $200 before we went back to our hotel for the evening.

I was just grateful to get an overnight experience with a long-time friend. I always wanted to do something like this with him, so I'm glad it worked out.

Kamikaze

It's always exciting to go on vacation, however, this trip was extra special because my uncle Gordon and aunt Theressa as they joined us at an all-inclusive. This was the first trip for my uncle going to an Island. We all stayed at the Royalton Punta Cana Resort and Casino, in 2017. Rick, Silvana, and Nick also joined us for fun in the sun in the D.R.

Gordon and Theressa arrived at what he referred to as "The Compound" later in the evening, since they flew with a different airline. We repeatedly explained to him that it was a resort and not some military base. It has tons of open space, beautiful landscaping, pools and a beach. We walked them around on our way to their room and my dad couldn't help but ask what Gordon thought of "The Compound." I knew that was coming, so I corrected him by reminding him it was a resort. We all laughed.

When they settled in, we took them to the Gourmet Marche-Buffet to grab some much overdue food as their five-hour flight had been delayed by forty-five minutes by a storm. Gordon couldn't believe how plentiful and delicious the food was at the buffet. I remember him saying that it was a "big eye-opener" and that he made the assumption that the food wouldn't be up to par.

A few days after Gordon had time to soak the island life in, he came back from a morning walk and said he was really enjoying the resort. He told Theressa he would love to do it every other year. All of us looked at each other, happy he was really enjoying himself because we were a little worried about how he would take it based on his attitude leading up to the vacation.

One afternoon, we made our way over to a water-park that was semi-attached to our resort to re-experience our childhoods. The park features a children's pool complete with water slides, a wave pool, as well as a selection of water tubes you can grab.

My dad asked one of the lifeguards how safe it would be for me to go down one of the slides. The lifeguard assumed that we were talking about the shortest slide and told us it was very safe as he pointed it out. My dad and I looked at each other, knowing that he misunderstood which slide we were talking about. "No, sir. How safe is the higher one?" my dad asked. The lifeguard looked and couldn't give a clear answer, but eventually said it was safe.

The Kamikaze Water Slide is a fifty-foot vertical drop, which is about seven stories high. After climbing all those stairs, I knew there was only one way down. Nick went down first followed by my dad. Stirling helped me get into position since I was next in line. I always say that if you're going to die while doing something you wanted to do, well, here's to life. I folded my arms across my chest and down I went, sliding faster than I could have imagined. My heart was beating out of my chest on the way down. I hit the water at the bottom and came to a quick stop. I loved it and wanted to try the higher slides.

While I was up there, I had a flashback to last year when Silvana freaked out when she saw me fall into the pool. Luckily, this episode was caught on film, so I can quote Silvana verbatim in all her panic. "Oh shit! Oh, oh, I think Kyle is coming down. Oh, the blue one. I think that's him up there. Oh my God. Should I close my eyes? Oh, dear. Oh, dear, that's Kyle. Ohhhh. Ohhhh. Ohhhhhhh. I know, my heart is racing!"

The next evening, an older Polish man came up to me and, in broken English, said, "You, great job up there. I watched you come down. I clapped for you."

Seven Fabulous Tens

My aunt Jean, who lives in Florida, has never been to an island before and has always talked about wanting to go to an all-inclusive with us. On her seventieth birthday, we finally made it happen. Rick, Silvana, Nick and my family left from Pearson Airport in Toronto as Aunt Jean and her niece, Kristen, left from Tampa Bay.

In 2018, we stayed at the Royalton Bavaro Resort and Spa in Punta Cana. When Jean and Kristen arrived an hour after us, we got our rooms, unpacked, and relaxed for a bit. Afterwards, we went to have some lunch.

We ate at the Score Bar and Lounge, which had a casual atmosphere. The rest of the afternoon was spent by the diamond pool drinking our "special drink" of the hour. "Woohoo, the week is finally here!" Jean said with excitement.

As we were all getting ready to have our first dinner at the Hunter Steakhouse, Jean and Kristen knocked on my parents' room and were a little early. My dad was dressed, but my mom was in the shower. I was in my own room next to my parents, but it was an adjoining room. "Kristen and I will sit out on the pool balcony," Jean told my dad, who decided to tag along. My dad misjudged the power needed to close the sliding door and his baby finger got caught; he saw stars. He said that he thought he was in Florida for a moment where the doors are often very difficult to close and muscle memory took over. Jean and Kristen heard the door slam but weren't aware of what happened, distracted by the beautiful scenery. My dad walked to the pool in front of them and gently put his baby finger in the swim out pool. As the conversation continued as nothing happened, Jean asked, shocked, if she saw blood in the pool.

As I wheeled into my parents' room, I noticed things were busy at the double sink. "Look what happened, Kyle," my dad said, wincing in pain. He raised his hand to show me before wrapping his baby finger with tape. "Well, at least it matches the other baby finger," I said sarcastically. His other baby finger had suffered a similar fate years earlier, that left physically altered and stunted growth. We ended up laughing it off and washed down the pain with some white wine at dinner.

On Jean's actual birthday (October 25th) or the "Seven Fabulous Tens Day" as she called it, we started the day at the Royal Spa after a celebration breakfast. Believe it or not, this was actually her first ever trip to a spa. That morning I woke up with a severe stiff neck and couldn't move. I booked a twenty-minute massage hoping to get some relief from the stiffness. We all met at the water therapy room to enjoy some quiet time. After the spa, we spent time in the Royalton Lazy River with a few special drinks. Later on, we went to our reservation at the Zen Teppanyaki and Sushi Bar. The chefs cooked everything right in front of us.

As we were leaving, they had a talented live band playing in the bar area. Jean loves dancing, so of course, she joined the crowd with my mom. A tall, handsome, young man with dreadlocks grabbed Jean and took her around the dance floor. After a few dances, he claimed she tired him out. "Not bad for turning seventy, eh?" my dad said to him. Dreadlocks was completely shocked and disappeared into the crowd.

Every night on our way back from dinner and spending time in the lobby, we would always stop by the Beach Bar in front of our rooms to have a few more drinks. However, I don't know what it was, but it was like our presence was needed to get the party rolling. Within ten minutes of us being there, the bar would become jammed packed. When the bartenders got to know us, they always looked forward to seeing us, especially Jean. One of the bartenders would let her take home the half-drunk chardonnay she would nurse because, as she would say, "You never throw out a bottle of wine until it's empty."

This trip was a huge improvement for our friend Silvana's fear of water. Last year, she brought a swimsuit and practised walking into the pool up to her ankles. It took a while, but we eventually got her in up to her neck, albeit with a lot of anxiety. We're all really proud of Silvana for attempting to overcome her fear.

However, we had a secret weapon that gave her the courage she needed to conquer her fear: *BOOZE*. Silvana loves her drinks, so if she wanted a drink, she had to get herself to the pool bar. And the only way she could get her margarita was to walk to the bar through the water. It was like dangling a carrot in front of a horse.

Rio Rodizio is located on the second floor of a building overlooking the Atlantic Ocean and the Caribbean Sea. Following a centuries-old tradition of cooking on an open fire, diners can experience endless cuts of succulent beef, pork, lamb and chicken carved tableside in the style of authentic Brazilian gauchos. A two-sided disk is used by diners to signal when they're ready for more sizzling skewers: green means more and red means we're good for now. You basically eat as much as you want at your own pace.

Getting into the restaurant had a few stairs. They built a steep ramp off the side for accessible entry. As we were leaving, my dad decided to play another prank on our friend, Silvana. He pretended to lose control of my wheelchair and I sped down the ramp like a *NASCAR* driver gunning it for the finish line. Silvana, who was standing at the bottom of the ramp, looked at me with fear in her eyes and began to scream, fearing I was about to crash into a wall. I just softly touched the wall, but no serious injuries. Poor Silvana, once again almost had a heart-attack.

Everyone truly enjoyed each other's company on this trip. We made new memories with Aunt Jean. Jean loved the trip and claimed it was the "Best birthday week ever!"

Wendel Goons

During one of my trips to Buffalo with Steven to see a Leafs-Sabres game, we saw a bunch of guys who dressed up as Leaf Goons who wore white helmets. Steven said, "Kyle, look over there. The Wendel Goons are here!" I guess they heard us because they made their way over to us. They saw that we were wearing Leafs jerseys and wanted to take a picture with us. Maybe it should have been the other way around, but we treated it like we were famous for something instead of the picture.

We finally got to our seats which had a perfect view of the ice, twenty rows up from the bottom, behind the Leafs' zone. Throughout the game, we were having great conversations and laughing with two Sabres fans sitting behind us.

The Leafs beat the Sabres 4-2 and the entire arena shook as everyone chanted, "GO, LEAFS, GO!" All the fans gave each other high fives over a great game and win.

Royalton Awaits Us...

It was the evening before another trip to Punta Cana. My uncle Gordon, aunt Theressa and my brother's girlfriend, Kerri, spent the night at our house so we could leave by three in the morning. We also picked up Rick, Silvana and their son Nick along the way to Toronto.

Two o'clock came quickly. Gordon and Theressa came back in after loading up the van, saying with trembling voices that it was cold outside. "Not for long," I said with a priceless smile.

Once we arrived at the Park 'n' Fly, Rick, Silvana and Nick met Kerri "Underwood" for the first time. She greeted them with a big smile and hug, which is something I love about her. She always greets everyone with a hug no matter who it is.

Toronto's Pearson Airport had changed their check-in systems over the years so they would be automated, effectively dropping human interaction to a minimum. The few staff who were on duty tried to guide my dad and me to the "special service" line to get me through faster. This is a good system for people with a disability or medical conditions, but not when you're with a large group like we were as they tried to separate us. They only wanted to let my dad and me through and leave the rest behind. The automated lines took twice as long, which begs the question of why they're even considered in the first place. Cost savings over customer convenience, I guess. When we made it through our line, we had to wait for everyone else before heading to the terminal.

Once we got on the plane, Stirling, Kerri and I sat together. Kerri asked if I was excited with a lot of excitement of her own in her voice. "For what?" I asked with a straight face. "Oh, shuuut uuup KYLE!" she responded in a high-pitched voice. Of course, I was excited, but I like messing with people.

When Kerri fell asleep on the airplane, she had her head down and her ponytail pointed up and back down like a swan's neck. She looked like a swan that was frozen by an evil villain or something. I couldn't help but laugh because that's all I could see when I looked over.

We finally arrived in Punta Cana after a forty-minute delay. In the years that we had been going down to Punta Cana, the airport had developed architecturally. Normally they had airstairs to get on and off the plane which was very inconvenient with my CP. This time, I noticed they had done away with the stairs and now had what's called an Aviramp — a combination of aviation ramp I guess? It's basically a properly graded ramp that slowly descends to the ground. Needless to say, it's so much easier for people with disabilities and every airport that doesn't have tunnel access should have these. These few modifications beats being carried up and down the stairs while sitting in an air transfer chair. Two men would be on either side of me and holding the bars on the sides of the chair. I would just trust and pray to God that one of them would not drop me or trip. That would be the end of my trip.

Once we got past Immigration to make sure we were who we said we were, we collected our luggage and hopped on a bus. Twenty minutes later, we arrived at the same resort as last year, The Royalton Bavaro. We picked this resort again because we knew Gordon and Theressa would enjoy it after our positive experience last year. We knew they were excited, hungry and ready to relax poolside. This was confirmed by Theressa when she said, "Boy, this is a bloody long walk to the Diamond Club!"

When we made it to our room, I was pleasantly surprised to find a green water float sitting in my swim out pool area. Green is my favourite colour; I even have green water shoes. If I can pick the colour of something, it's going to be green. The float itself might have blown off someone else's balcony and into mine, but I wasn't going to question where it came from. I knew this was going to be a fun trip after that little surprise.

After getting some food in our bellies, my dad, Theressa, and I hit the pool near the beachfront. My dad and I ordered our favourite cocktail called the Dirty Monkey while Theressa got a frozen margarita before hopping into the crystal-clear pool for some conversation.

Theressa mentioned that she recently saw a YouTube video of an English fellow who married an able-bodied woman who was his physician assistant. "See, there's hope Kyle," she said. "It just takes that one special woman to see past your CP." She had said something like this before to me, but with that enormous margarita in her hand, I told her she was just drunk. Although she claimed she wasn't, I couldn't resist the opportunity to tease her!

We booked the Oceanside Seafood Restaurant for dinner on the first night. The restaurant is located only several feet away from the beach, with its glass curtain walls, enjoying great views of the sunset. Gordon and Theressa went for a beautiful walk around the resort before meeting us at the restaurant. As I approached, I could hear Theressa say that they didn't have us down for our reservation and couldn't take us. My parents were perplexed because Diamond Club members have their reservations taken care of by the staff directly. It turns out that when you're ten or more people, reservations can't be made. Large groups become what's called "Family Style," which means platters of food are brought to the table instead of having them order off the menu. We really didn't understand how one more person made a difference, but we went along with it.

They immediately brought out appetizer platters and my mom mentioned that Stirling was celebrating his twenty-fourth birthday, to which the waiter said, "No problemo. We will make it special!" The food was very delicious. They served steaks, sausages, lamb, lobster and shrimp, with potatoes, rice, and vegetables. Am I making you hungry yet?

Once we finished up our plates, the staff started singing "Happy Birthday" in Spanish for Stirling, who wasn't at the table at the time. The staff paused as our waiter was signing to stop from across the room. Everyone started to laugh and our waiter asked where Stirling went. We all said, "Baño," which is a bathroom in Spanish. With Stirling making his way back to the table and completely oblivious to what had happened while he was away, the staff came out to try again. Before we left, I let everyone know that Kerri was picking up the bill for us — gotta keep the Scott traditions alive for the newest member of the family.

Every morning, I would get up around 7:00 a.m. to have a swim before breakfast. I noticed that the green water float was still there, so I figured I would take it for a ride. I met one of our neighbours while floating around who happened to be from Mississauga, about thirty minutes from Hamilton. I remember her stating that I looked comfortable in my float. My dad explained how we happened upon it the day before. The lady said, "Funny thing is that since we arrived four days ago, we have been the only ones here and that float has been visiting all of our pool areas." I guess I was just the lucky one the day before, so I called the float my "Gift from Heaven."

Later on in the morning, Gordon took me to the pool for a little freedom in the water. Since my dang hip doesn't cooperate and it's extremely difficult to walk independently, Gordon was helping me get in. However, I decided to take the most difficult way down to cause a spectacle. We both walked down the steps with a railing between us and as I got further down, I decided to go under the railing. Gordon grabbed my ankles to get my feet back on solid ground on the other side. I slipped through, went under the water, and popped back to say, "I thought it was the easiest way to get in!" The people watching were amazed by such a dramatic and unnecessary entrance into the pool. Gordon and I had a good laugh over the theatrics.

At some point, we met this lovely young retired couple from Barrie (about an hour and a half from Hamilton) who had recently moved to Scotland. While engaged in conversation, a butterfly landed on my head that I didn't notice. My mom actually pointed it out to me. Now, ever since my grandma Scott (Evelyn) passed away, I had been running into a lot of butterflies. I always associated them with her, so I felt like it was her doing. For instance, during the previous summer, our backyard filled with butterflies. I believe it's her watching over us and letting us know she's there.

Everyone around was amazed, including the Canadian/Scottish couple, because when does something like that ever happen? The butterfly was a beautiful light brown with golden trim along with the wings and it had to land on my perfectly shaped head. This butterfly, or should I say, Grandma, sat on my head for a good few minutes before any of us thought of taking a picture. Thankfully it stayed there long enough for its photo opportunity.

The following day, most of us wanted to relax in the Royalton Lazy River that is over 1,200 feet long. Theressa and my mom paired up in this big, blue cube that could only hold two people like my dad and I followed behind them. My mom didn't ride the river the previous year and didn't know what to expect. My aunt gave her the full experience, making sure she went under every waterfall we drifted by.

While I was passing through one of the more powerful waterfalls — and they feel great, by the way, if you have neck and back issues, a perfect way to relax your muscles — I noticed Kerri was looking for us as she were further away. Stirling wasn't with her either because he tends to wander off and does his own thing sometimes. I asked her where my brother was. She thought he would be with us, which he wasn't. She asked me if I wanted to float around with her instead, but I told her that I wasn't responsible for anything that could happen like driving straight into a waterfall, which we did, but she got me back by grabbing my ankles in an attempt at being a baby shark. Like anyone would believe a shark would be in the lazy river. Kerri, you have such an imagination.

In the middle of our "Royalton life" vacation I got up early for my morning routine. Outside in the swim out pool, my dad and our Canadian neighbours noticed a big, ugly cloud covering the resort. It didn't take long for the first signs of rain to present itself. My dad and I figured we would just stay in since we were wet anyway. Kra-koom! A streak of lightning convinced us pretty quick to get out, so we hightailed it out of there lickety-split. As we got out to dry off a bit before we went to the lobby for breakfast, the phone rang. Sunwing Airlines called to discuss a few issues that we were having, specifically screwing up our rooms, which seems to happen every year with these guys. They always promise that the next visit will be special to make up for it, but it never happens. They don't know how to solve a problem, but can surely take your money in a flash. Dad and I stayed behind and let everyone go on ahead. Once off the phone, the weather basically turned into a tropical storm, leaving us trapped in the room since we would need to walk for about five minutes out in the open. We let everyone know via text that we were going to the Diamond Club area, which was in the same building, to eat instead.

After about an hour, the rain began to slow down enough for us to make a beeline for the rest of our group. There they were lounging around, having their morning drinks and relaxing. Theressa told us that Gordon and she had been there since 7:00 a.m. because when they woke up, the clock was ahead by an hour. They didn't understand why the resort was empty until they saw the actual time on the lobby clock. They assumed most people sleep in while on the resort. "I was up," I told her. "I was just taking a shit though!" She almost fell to the ground from laughing so hard.

Since the weather wasn't cooperating that day, we decided to have a spa day. The men and women were split up into two groups at this point. One of the first things we were asked to do was get into ice-cold water to close our pores, which isn't relaxing whatsoever. You're in the sun all day and then told to jump into a -40 degrees lake to close your pores — talk about rigor mortis. Afterwards, we went straight into a sauna for ten minutes. It was about 60 degrees Celsius at first, but by the end of it, it was somewhere around 71 to 93 degrees. We couldn't stand it and had to get out; we were on fire. We went into a different one that was no better temperature-wise, but it had eucalyptus mixed in with the steam.

After twenty minutes of popping in and out of saunas, we joined back up with the ladies and were brought to the hydrotherapy room, which is basically just jets of water blasted over your body. We laid down with cucumbers on our eyes and relaxed for about ten minutes. I have to say that was the most relaxing part of the entire vacation and, no, we didn't eat the cucumbers.

Sadly, our vacation came to an end, but only until our next one. Everything was going smoothly until I was singled out and placed under investigation. My wheelchair was considered a possible risk for stowing away contraband. I was amused by the experience of being frisked down, while every eye in the airport was on me. Our group thought it was hilarious but I didn't hold it against airport security because they have a job to do.

Once I was all clear, Gordon said, "Travelling today is harder than years ago, but they might have thought that you looked like a criminal."

Kerri finished off that thought by adding, "Yeah, Kyle, you're dangerous!" I definitely felt the love and support of my family that day.

While we were waiting at the terminal, we noticed that our flight time was fast approaching. Normally, those needing assistance are boarded first. My dad and I went up to the staff to make sure they knew we needed help. Thankfully we did because they had no clue. With many apologies, they made the necessary arrangements, gathered everyone needing assistance, and took us to the tarmac. For five minutes, we stood there in blistering

38-degree heat; the sun roasted us from above, while the tarmac melted our shoes. A bus eventually arrived to transport us to the plane, but the airport associates, let all the able-bodied people on first and drove off. I'm not even joking, all of the disabled passengers and those needing help walked, WALKED, to the plane on their own. It was totally ridiculous and I don't know how anyone couldn't see what was wrong with this picture. You could clearly see we needed help!

After that fiasco, we finally got on the plane. An airport assistant sat me in a chair and brought me up backwards into the plane after my mom told them beforehand that it would be a lot easier to leave me in my wheelchair and wheel me up the ramp. Remember that old saying, "You can lead a horse to water?" A prime example if there ever was one.

An hour and thirteen minutes later and we were still on the tarmac. The pilot announced that we couldn't fly because of the weight of the plane and asked us all to get off. So, everybody groaned and got off. The pilot eventually received the okay to fly after they figured out how to shed some weight in the luggage, which meant we all had to pile back in to finally get home.

An hour into the flight, a flight attendant asked if there were any nurses or doctors on board. My aunt Theressa is an ICU nurse, so she volunteered. They came to the conclusion that the gentleman had the stomach flu, so they did what they could, which wasn't much, and made him comfortable for the rest of the flight.

While landing, Sunwing told us that some of the luggage was left behind. We were all praying that ours made it because we didn't want to spend any more time on this trip than was necessary. Thankfully our prayers were heard and we got everything we took with us. Despite the hiccups on the way home, everyone really enjoyed themselves and their time in the sun.

Chapter 12: Amusing Anecdotes

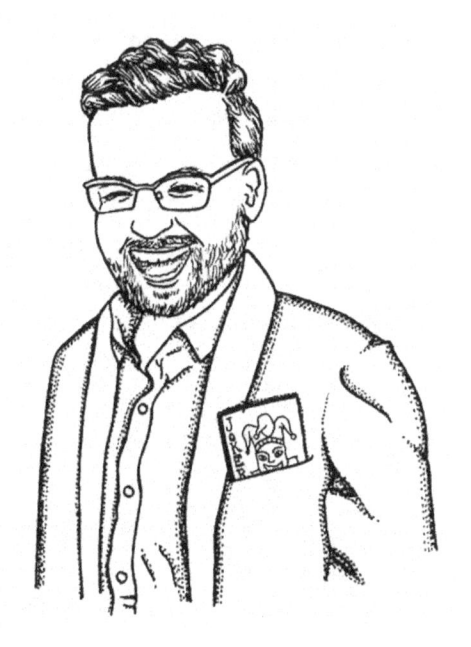

Stupidman and Lois Leak

When Mom was pregnant and had my brother Stirling, a client of my dad's named Laura helped me while he was working evenings at the salon. Laura has two grown daughters, who were in their mid-teens at the time, and a husband named Glen.

Laura is most certainly an entertaining person, and by that, I mean a drama queen. She can turn a molehill into a mountain by embellishing any story just to catch your attention. I say this in a loving way. She really is a very caring and generous person who would give you the shirt off her back in a second... well, maybe three seconds. She has a hard time lifting her arms due to an autoimmune disorder.

When my brother Stirling was a year and a half old, he couldn't pronounce Laura's name. Stirling would call her "Ya-Ya" instead. Laura thought that was just great, so she insisted she was called Ya-Ya while her husband took on the name "Mr. Pizza" instead of Mr. Peace. Why Mr. Pizza, you ask? A very common and easy first word for kids is pizza, so it made sense to pick something simple for us to latch on to.

When Ya-Ya started taking care of me, we would play floor hockey every day. All of the sounds of the rink could be heard in the living room where we played. I would play on my knees and in a position that allowed me to scoot side to side for the best mobility. One day, after two months of playing professional floor hockey, the ball rolled away from the living room "rink." To Laura's surprise, I got up and walked to get it, laughing the whole time I did it. Ya-Ya was shocked and had no idea that I could walk.

She asked my parents why I wasn't on my feet more. My parents were very concerned about broken bones if I were to fall, but they finally agreed that the game would be more fulfilling if I were on my feet and practising my mobility.

In the warmer months, we took our play outside where we would pretend to be "Stupidman" and "Lois Leak," a hopeless couple of dud superheroes who could never quite save the day. Stupidman could not remember what he was flying off to do most of the time and Lois Leak ran away from the emergency because she would always have to pee. I made sure Ya-Ya always got a good workout doing double duty as she flew me around the yard, my fake cape flapping in the wind.

Unfortunately, we had a very curious yet unfriendly neighbour at the time. When I was out playing with Ya-Ya, he would stand across the street staring at us. One time, I waved and said, "Hello," but he just sneered and continued to stare. Ya-Ya was very angry and had enough. She decided to keep us waving at him for a half-hour until he eventually went into the house. Victorious, Ya-Ya scoffed, "Good! Now we can play in a more pleasant environment," as we went back to playing Stupidman and Lois Leak.

A Yawn Way Down

Ya-Ya continued to look after me once school was done for the day to help assist with tasks like getting off the bus, bathroom duties, and playtime. One day after I got home from school, I ran to the bathroom because I needed to pee unbelievably bad. Ya-Ya was sitting on the edge of the tub waiting for me to do my business. Looking the other way, she wasn't expecting what was going to happen next. I took a big yawn, fully extending my arms, and accidentally knocked her into the tub. She fell backwards with her arms grasping at the air and legs flung up in a "V" shape. Stunned, Ya-Ya asked for my help, but what was I supposed to do? I looked down at her and coldly said, "Nope," and started laughing. Ever the drama queen, Ya-Ya, kicked and thrashed around like a fish, trying to get herself upright. She eventually did, without injury by the way, but I was in tears laughing my head off at something I would never forget. Here we are decades later and it's in my book!

Check One, Two, Flush

One of the worst times in my life has been going for a hearing test and, wouldn't you know it, they discovered I have high pitch hearing loss. What? What? It turned out that I needed hearing aids. Boy, was I ever against getting them. I fought every day, trying to get my educational assistant, Mrs. Gould, to take them out. At the time, I understood why I needed them, but it was way too loud, especially for a kid. I wore them for a few hours a day during school, just never at home. Once my speech therapist found out about the hearing loss and the hearing aids, they decided to take away my speech therapy. My parents were furious at the decision of taking the speech therapy away completely because it made no sense when I have speech dysarthria (slurred or slowed speech). The theory given was that the hearing aids would solve all my problems because they said that my speech would improve with the hearing aids. I think they lost a few steps in their program, they forgot that I had cerebral palsy, and my nerves and muscles were involved in my hearing loss, and also my speech.

    I became very frustrated and angry having to deal with hearing aids because I had a hard time adjusting to them. My parents fought tooth and nail over it, but the therapist wouldn't budge. If we knew a hearing test was going to result in the loss of speech therapy, my parents wouldn't have allowed it to happen. Now keep in mind that hearing aids have come a long way over the decades, so they're a lot better today than they were, but back then they were a disaster.

    After a few months of having these things, I was at my wit's end. I went to the school washroom one day to change my t-shirt with the help of Mrs. Gould. Not thinking about the hearing aids, the t-shirt somehow caught my ear and ripped one-off, sending it right into the toilet. I quickly looked at Mrs. Gould and asked without hesitating if I could flush it down. The poor woman had this worried look on her face because she thought the water had damaged it. Meanwhile, I wasn't worried at all and was actually excited at the prospect of never wearing them again. Mrs. Gould scooped it out of the toilet, rinsed it off, and used a paper towel to dry it off. She later put it in rice to try to soak up the excess moisture and wouldn't you know, the darn thing still worked. I was disappointed, but I probably would have had to get another one anyway, and the cost of them is nothing to scoff at. When my parents heard about the incident, they were cool with it, but if only they could have seen how panicked Mrs. Gould was at the time. It scared the living wits out of her thinking she might have made a mistake that would cost thousands to fix.

Gravity Hurts

In grade four, we had the pleasure — or displeasure, depending on how you look at it — of having our classroom in a portable several feet from the school's back doors. Portables aren't the quietest place for a classroom because it's basically a box elevated off the ground and it would be a little too loud since I wore hearing aids. The teacher for the class, Mrs. Mooney, had the brilliant idea of using tennis balls on the bottom of our chairs to lower the noise for me. The hearing aids that I wore picked up every little sound at twice the volume it should have.

One particular day while Mrs. Mooney was teaching, a massive bang happened at the back of the classroom. Everyone jerked around to see what the heck happened and there was Ryan, our class joker, laying flat out on the floor with his desk, books, and other items covering his body. Ryan loved rocking his chair back, but this time he lost his balance. One of the classmates yelled out exactly what everyone was thinking: "Finally!"

In gym class, we would often play dodgeball. I was going backwards, keeping my eyes on the ball so I wouldn't get "tagged out." I didn't know that one of my classmates was down on the floor behind me while I was backing up and I ended up tripping over my classmate Gregg. Down I went, falling backwards and hitting my head on the floor. I actually saw stars and felt dazed.

While Gregg was trying to help me up, he knew that I was unconscious and yelled out for help. After laying on the gym floor for a few minutes, I looked up and said, "Am I out?" I wanted to continue playing despite being sent for a loop. Mrs. Gould took me to the staff room to put some ice on my head and to make sure I didn't fall asleep in case I had a concussion. Turned out that I had a concussion.

Mrs. Gould called my dad to explain the incident. My dad was waiting for me to come home and when I got there, he noticed a huge lump on my head and put more ice on it. One of my dad's clients who worked at a hospital said to keep a close eye on me and to look out for any nausea or confusion. I ended up being okay and only suffered from the lump and a headache in the end.

Rodent You Know It

On one sunny Saturday afternoon, I decided to play hockey in the backyard by myself with a street hockey goalie set placed on pieces of wood. I was getting hungry and while I was trying to open the door back into the house, I saw a chipmunk running under my feet. In my mind, I thought for sure that it was going to run up my leg. Freaking out a little bit, I pulled on the handle several times, and wouldn't you know it, I couldn't get it open.

I couldn't see where the chipmunk went. Panic set in and I lost my footing and, of course, down I went with my head striking the wrought-iron railings. Lunch was on hold and off I went to what seemed like my second home, the hospital, to have staples put into my head. The doctor asked me how this happened and seconds earlier I happened to notice a calendar hanging on the wall that had a chipmunk on the top. I pointed out the chipmunk and explained what had happened. After a good laugh, the doctor said it was the first time he had to give someone staples because of a chipmunk.

Onion Tossers

On one Monday afternoon, Ya-Ya, my dad and I were at Montana's BBQ and Bar for lunch. Ya-Ya ordered a burger that came with onions. She wanted to eat them but didn't want the stinking breath because she was going to a dinner function with her husband Glen. The only solution was a game of ring toss.

My dad put his nose up in the air to act as the post. Ya-Ya tried her best but threw the onion into a lady's hair behind my dad. The lady turned around like she was going to kill us, but saw that I was laughing so hard that I was gasping for air. She must have thought I had done it by accident, so she smiled, nodded, and went back to her lunch. Relieved at avoiding drama, Ya-Ya said, "Thanks for taking one for the team, Kyle!"

Soak Up the Sun

My uncle Brian and aunt Anna took James and me to one of the autumn fairs in our area. James and I went on this ride that looked like a flying saucer spaceship that belongs to the NASA training facility. We were standing upright against a padded wall and it did what it was supposed to do, spin like crazy. Poor James has never felt more sick and nauseous in his life. He came out of there totally messed up.

On our way home, we spent the entire ride in the back of Anna and Brian's four-door with James looking two steps from vomiting everywhere. There wasn't much I could do to help out his spins, but I know that day that I had a great friend in James. If anyone stuck around with my crazy aunt Anna, who played Sheryl Crow's "Soak Up the Sun" on repeat a million times, while holding back his breakfast, he's a friend for life.

Hiding Undie the Tree

During the summer of 2003, Ya-Ya wanted to take me out to celebrate after graduating from grade eight, so we went for lunch and a movie date. When it was all over and we got back into Ya-Ya's car, I noticed an old pair of underwear that was lying in the back seat. When I pointed them out, she claimed that she was looking for the same style and brought them with her into stores as reference.

Ya-Ya then jumped out of the car and ran up to the closest tree while screaming "Toxic waste!" I seriously thought she had lost her mind. She cocked her arm back and chucked the undies into the tree, catching perfectly at the end of a branch. It took everything in me to not pee myself laughing as we sped off down the road.

Elite Golfers Only

My mom has a very large and close Italian family. It's not uncommon for us to have a ton of different gatherings throughout the year. During the summer of 2004, my great-uncle Tony and aunt Felicia hosted a summer party at their big property in Caledonia, Ontario. Just a quick note: Great-Uncle Tony shouldn't be confused with my mom's brother Tony, the same Tony who has been an inspiration to me and whom I have spoken about previously in this book. We're an Italian family so you have to expect a few Tonys here and there.

Anyway, the morning after the party, we wanted to properly thank them for a fun outing but my dad wanted to play a prank on them. My dad called pretending to be the owner of the Sunset Driving Range located directly across the street from my great-uncle's house. Tony picks up and is immediately asked if he would be interested in selling his property for $5 million so they could expand their business by creating an entire golf course for "elite golfers." My dad also offered to hire Tony as the head mechanic for the carts. Cha-ching! Tony had money signs in his eyes. "Talk it over with your wife," my dad said, but Tony's response was, "Oh no, I'm going to tell her, 'Too bad!' I can give her half and she can divorce me. *Fanculo* [f**k off in Italian] if she doesn't like it." (He said this in a typical Italian, loving way.)

My dad had him going as he was clearly on cloud nine, thinking he had hit the big time. I would even jokingly go as far as to say that Tony would throw anyone under the bus just to get a piece of that money. In the background, you could hear his wife calming him down because he was getting so hyped up. The joke had its moment and we had to bring him down gently. We asked him if he knew someone named Kyle Scott. At first, he either didn't hear what was said or actually drew a blank, but then he went, "Oh, yeah, yeah. He's my great-nephew..." After a bit of pause, Tony finally processed what happened and gave out a roaring laugh on the phone. "You got me! You really got me!"

His wife was dying of laughing in the background, too, because she wasn't buying it but had seen how bright her husband's eyes were at the prospect of making an easy $5 million. "Really? Get a grip, Tony," she said to him. "Who in their right mind would call up and offer five million like that? Are you nuts?"

Having a family that spends time celebrating together whether it's a birthday, anniversary, wedding or just a simple gathering is truly a blessing and I love this part of my life.

Laying the Smackdown

As I've mentioned, professional wrestling runs quite deep in my family. My great-uncles George and Sandy (a.k.a. Angus) Scott were famous wrestlers, winning multiple Tag Team Champions under the name "The Flying Scott's" in the 1950s. In George's career, he had 1,519 matches from 1950-1981 with ring names, Benny Backer, George Scott, The Flying Scott's and

Amusing Anecdotes

The Great Scott. After retiring, he began working for Vince McMahon Sr. in the World Wide Wrestling Federation, known as (WWWF). With time, he also worked for Vince's son, Vince Jr., in the renamed World Wrestling Federation (WWF) in the '80s. As of 2002, the organization is known as World Wrestling Entertainment (WWE).

In 1983, Vince McMahon hired George as his chief booker, where he helped formulate WrestleMania 1 in 1985 in New York. The event featured names like Muhammad Ali as a guest referee, Liberace doing leg kicks with the Rockettes, and Mr. T teaming up with Hulk Hogan to take on Rowdy Roddy Piper and Paul Orndorff in the final bout. Vince told George, "If this thing doesn't work, we're bankrupt. We're going to have to close the company."

Within a few years, it was McMahon's competitors who were closing up shop. George and Vince Jr. followed up in 1986 with WrestleMania 2, featuring the recently retired Jesse Ventura, in whom George saw a perfect candidate with a furious personality that would spark a fire if needed, which enabled him to become a great commentator. He also invented the reversal to the "Nature Boy" Ric Flair's Figure-Four Leglock in the 1980's, where the opponent would simply turn over onto their stomach. Needless to say, our family loves professional wrestling and has traditions built around its legacy.

My uncle Gordon, Stirling, Dad and I often went to the movie theatre to watch the pay per view (PPV) wrestling events like the Royal Rumble and WrestleMania. We always bumped into the husband and son of one of my dad's hair salon clients, Mike Sr. and Mike Jr, both of whom are characters who also love wrestling. Mike Jr. is twelve years older than me and also has cerebral palsy that is considered extreme compared to my own.

Mike Sr. and I always wrestle when we see each other. I tend to sit behind him in the theatre, so I can get an advantage in the inevitable fight. I would cuff him from behind and pretended it was the person sitting next to me. He would get up, grab me by the t-shirt and pull me over into their row so he could beat the hell out of me in front of everyone. For dramatic effect, he would rip his cheap t-shirts half off and claim that it was me. Okay... I might have participated a little.

At one PPV, we made our match a street fight, which basically means it's outside of a building. I was trying to get into the van, but he was after me. He snuck up behind, putting me in a headlock. I gave him a punch to the head and quickly hopped into the van. He was unrelenting and followed me into the van. I booted him out and quickly slammed the sliding door on him. Mike Sr. tripped over the curb as he was reeling from my boot and crashed onto the sidewalk. When he got back up, he gave me the finger and pulled his pants down in defeat. It was a full moon I'll never forget.

My absolute favourite fight took place one year at the biggest show of them all, WrestleMania. We met the two Mikes and the rest of the group in the parking lot before heading in. As we passed the first set of French doors, Mike Sr. quickly shut the doors behind us before reaching the next set in an attempt to lock me in. The beating commenced and we clobbered each other all around that entryway. I tore Mike's pre-ripped shirt during the struggle, which he wore purposely for dramatic effect. He tipped my wheelchair over while still pounding me and we both fell to the floor in what probably looked like slow motion. We continued laying the smackdown until one of the theatre staff, who has seen us do this countless times, ran out pretending like we were actually fighting. Both of us immediately stopped to look at this guy who had a bit of fear in his eyes. "Every time you guys come here, you're always fighting," he proclaimed. "I'm going to have to report you guys to my manager this time."

Stand Away from This Man

It had been a few years since Ya-Ya and I had enjoyed one of our traditional lunch and movie dates in the spring of 2008. We went to our usual spot, Montana's, and walked over to the movie theatre afterwards. There was a middle-aged woman working at Cineplex and she always greeted me by saying, "Are you seeing a wee little movie today, sweetheart?"

Ya-Ya didn't take kindly to this and told the lady off before giving a huge eye roll. "Ma'am, speak to him as an intelligent twenty-year-old, not like he's three!" Ya-Ya always treated me like every other person and she felt it was disrespectful for anyone to treat someone like me any different.

After the movie, I was transferring from the theatre chair to my wheelchair and the same lady rushed in to help lift me up. Ya-Ya asked her not to touch me and explained that I had to find my own point of balance. The woman was being overly helpful and kept interfering. After three polite attempts at trying to get the woman to back down, Ya-Ya bellowed, "Stand away from this man!" The poor woman took off in a shot while I had myself a good laugh.

The one thing that you are assured of when you're in the presence of Ya-Ya, you just never know what to expect at any given moment but you will for sure be entertained.

What is a Hockey Legend Doing Here?

My dad and I went to a cousin's stag one Friday evening in June 2013. We found ourselves standing around talking when my cousin Mark came up to introduce someone to us. I knew who it was right away so we shook hands and exchanged pleasantries, while everyone else had huge smiles on their faces and laughing. My dad was confused and asked if we knew each other. "Dad, it's Doug Gilmour. He's a retired Toronto Maple Leafs legend," I proclaimed. My dad recognized him as someone, even saying he thought it might have been Doug, but questioned why he would be at the stag. My cousin's fiancé is a Leafs fan so it made sense to the rest of us.

Doug Gilmour was one of my favourite players as a kid. Unfortunately, when I went to the game and met the Leafs players at the Maple Leaf Garden in 1998, he had been traded to the New Jersey Devils a year prior. It was a great moment to finally get to meet one of my childhood heroes.

Gambling Man

I'm a gambler, I must admit. It all started when I was a bit younger (of course, I had to be legal age of nineteen) during one of our first visits to the Fallsview Casino in Niagara Falls. One of my mother's cousins showed us the perks of having a membership and explained that if you play at the casino, you will get free parking, dinner, and tickets to shows. We found this to be a great source of entertainment for the money and decided to give it a shot. I immediately fell in love, or maybe it was just addiction, with the excitement of winning. However, I hated losing, so we came up with the strategy of never putting our winnings back into the machine. You go in with a set amount of money, spend it and run off with your winnings. I was also attracted to the fact that I have independence on the machines since the buttons are big and I can pull the slot machine arms. It's always a fun night out with friends and family.

There was one instance that has stayed with me during my gambling career. While at the Niagara Falls Casino, I was playing a Wheel of Fortune machine. The guy next to me got a lucky spin but didn't win much. A minute later, he got another spin. He turned to me before spinning and said, "I haven't had much luck tonight. Would you like to hit it for me?" I was down, so I spun it for him. Around it went and as it began to slow down, it was getting awfully close to the grand prize. Wouldn't you know it, it landed on the highest amount possible, $1,000. I was actually thrilled to have been the person to win him a bit of money. The gentleman thanked me and gave me $100 out of the winnings. It was very generous of him to do that and I wasn't expecting it.

In everyone's lifetime, we often cross paths with extraordinary people. When someone does something nice or gives you something, it means you've formed a bond. This is what I call paying it forward. When someone inspires you, makes you feel good, or goes out of their way for you, maybe go out of your own way in return by buying them a drink or doing some other kind of gesture to pay forward their kindness.

Missing the Tip

We were invited to my second cousin Lucy's surprise sixtieth birthday party in April 2015. My dad and I were introduced to a man from Ireland who was a friend of the family. My dad asked him if he was taking Spanish lessons yet because his wife's family is from Argentina. The guy shook his head with a little laugh saying no.

"I would rethink that if I were you," my dad advised. "I didn't take Italian lessons right away like I promised I would for my wife." My dad lifted his baby finger to show him that something was wrong with it.

I knew where my dad was going with this joke and started to laugh. "It took me fourteen years, but they took this from me," he said, flashing his baby finger that's missing a bit from the tip (as I mentioned in the previous chapter). My dad proceeded to tell him that they took him to a basement and chopped it off. The Irishman had a completely blank face, unsure of how to respond. My dad's finger actually got caught in a door when he was a kid, so it's a little shorter from the accident. Before the guy could gather himself, my dad pointed to me and said, "And he used to be able to walk!" I almost fell out of my wheelchair from laughing so hard.

Little Natalie

In January 2017, my parents and I were at Wally-Mart (Wal-Mart) to return an item. While in line, I was watching this little girl helping her mom put items in the shopping cart. A while later, we saw the same girl at the in-store McDonald's. The girl came up to my mom and asked why I was in a wheelchair. My mom explained my disability to her. We found out that her name was Natalie and she was four years old. She sat with me for a bit and said I was a funny guy.

As they were leaving, Natalie came up to me and gave me a big hug, and said, "I hope you feel better!" Ten minutes later, as we were leaving, Natalie and her family were waiting for her mom to bring the van to the front of the store. Natalie came up to give me one more hug before she left, which was really cute and nice.

Natalie stole my heart after meeting with her and found out she lost a brother who was only two years old due to SIDS. I will never forget her infectious spirit, her compassion towards me and how she took the time to talk to me. So untouched by the world, but so wise beyond her years. She made my day a better day.

Kyle N. Scott

Pigskin Pete

One early afternoon in April 2019, my mom took our dog, Pepie, for a walk with two of our neighbours. While coming back, my mom noticed there was a sign on one of our neighbour's lawns, and initially thought their house was up for sale. In actuality, it said to vote for Kyle Scott as the next Pigskin Pete, (leads the Tiger-Cats fans in the traditional Oskee Wee Wee chant while wearing a custom number 6 Tiger-Cats jersey and a bowler hat) of the Hamilton Tiger-Cats football team. My mom was confused to see my name and asked the neighbour why she had my name on the sign. Neither my mom nor the neighbour knew that they each had a son with the same exact same name and that we lived seconds away from each other.

From that day on, I received texts from neighbours asking why they didn't know I applied to be Pigskin Pete. I just told everyone it was a secret and that I was disappointed it was out of the bag. This thing was even in the local *Mountain News* newspaper. When I found that out, I harassed my mom to dig through the recycling. She wouldn't do it until I told her "I" was in it.

My mom took a photo of the sign and I posted it on Facebook with the caption, "Well, I am now living the dream of being Pigskin Pete!" Within a few minutes, everybody was hitting the like, love, and laugh buttons and commenting "Congrats," thinking it was me. The next morning, people began to realize it wasn't actually me, so the jig was up, but I wasn't going to let this thing die. So, I reached out to the other Kyle Scott to let him know what I was up to.

"Congratulations Kyle, from another Kyle Scott on Hamilton's mountain," I said in a message to him. "I have been riding your coattails in your journey to becoming the next Pigskin Pete. I have had numerous emails in congratulatory response to what they think is me running for Pigskin Pete. The straw that broke the camel's back was your picture in the *Mountain News*. Thanks for the unexpected laughs I had with friends and family while I stole a bit of your spotlight. With a name like ours, it sounds like a sure win. All the best, enjoy the ride. I'm thirty-years-old and have cerebral palsy, so I use a wheelchair at this point, and thought it was funny imagining my fan base wondering how I was going to be a mascot. You have my vote, and many others!"

Within a few minutes, the other Kyle replied, "That is absolutely amazing. What a story. Can you tag me on Facebook? Man, that's absolutely awesome, and would love to meet you one day."

To show my support, I offered to buy one of his t-shirts and have his sign on our lawn. He asked where I was located. Little did we know that my neighbours a few houses down was his mom. He came over personally to meet me and gave me a t-shirt. We took pictures to share the story with everyone, too, and posted them on Facebook.

From that moment on, I asked all my friends and family to vote for my "name twin," which probably got him a few hundred more votes, some of which came in from the States. We stayed in communication and he was very thankful for all the support. He didn't do too bad in the votes, but he was decidedly edged out by someone else by quite a few votes. I wanted a recount because it seemed fishy, but I selfishly only really wanted to have my name associated with the Tiger-Cats and Pigskin Pete.

Chapter 13: With Us in Spirit: Tributes to Family and Friends Who Have Passed

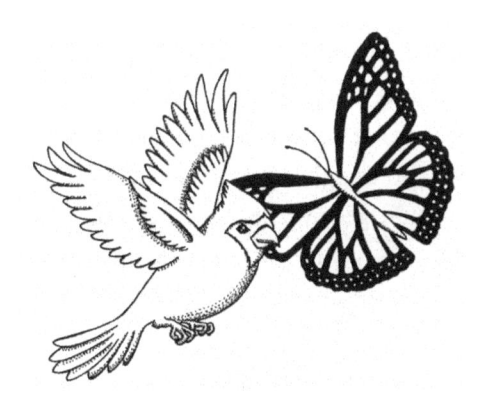

Jovial Nonno

On Tuesday, April 30th, 1996, my nonno Nicola D'Agostino passed away at the age of seventy-one after battling lung cancer. Even though I was blessed to have him in my life for six years, he was the first major loss that I suffered.

I often went to visit and spend time with him; I remember bringing him a "Get Well" card that I made. While visiting one time, my nonno said, "That damn disability!"

My dad asked if he was talking about my CP, which Nonno confirmed. "Dad, Kyle is fine and well looked after. You need to get better because we need your help," my dad told him in response. My nonno was worried about me and his wife right up until the end. I remember him asking my dad to take care of his wife, Maria, when he was gone, which we absolutely did.

I would see my nonno and nonna several times a week. Nonno would pick me up every day from school to bring me to their house until my parents could bring me home. My nonni (grandparents) would always do thoughtful things for us, usually pertaining to food, like when my nonna would make homemade pizzas and bring them over to our place for dinners. After several unexpected pizza visits, my parents were like "You just brought pizza yesterday!"

My nonno would say, "I know. I just want to see my mazzamauriello." A mazzamauriello is basically a puppet on strings that are attached to woodblocks. This was his nickname for me; I was his little puppet.

My nonno would do anything to make sure I was happy and would go to great lengths to ensure it. He drove a Pontiac and each time I rode in it, I would get motion sick. He believed that it was the car that was making me sick, so he went out and bought a brand-new car. Isn't that a true showing of love? I think I would get overheated in the car, because he never put the windows down, and would get overwhelmed by it all. He must have been afraid of me getting a draft in 27 degrees Celsius weather. God bless that man.

Nonno was a very hard-working construction worker for more than thirty years. He was a member of the Fondi Club that was created by family and friends who came from Italy. He was a very patient person who loved life, food, and his family. He had a jovial sense of humour and was a jokester like most of us are, and he also loved to help where he could. He danced with everyone, especially his wife and my mom, and was a great person who was very respected by everyone who knew him. We all miss you, Nonno, and I know you're watching us from up above.

Gone So Young, Too Soon

Our family was struck another heavy blow that same year when my uncle Kevin passed away on Friday, August 9th, 1996. He was only thirty-one years old when he lost his battle against cancer after fighting for two and a half years.

I remember my grandpa Scott being devastated by the loss. It took him about three years to kind of come out of his spell a little bit. He suffered from really bad depression during that time, which was confirmed in a diary the family found years later after his own passing. He wrote about the emotional toll it took on him as a father to lose one of his sons at such a young age.

I remember when Kevin used to tease my cousin Brittany and me. He would say random and funny things like, "You stink! Go and take a bath!"

Kevin was the tallest in the family at 6'4". He was a hard worker who loved cars and worked as a detailer at Johnson Chrysler on Upper James in Hamilton. He had the incredible ability of being able to pick up a language very quickly, such as Polish, Korean and some Italian.

He was a very private person, but gentle with those around him, especially his parents and his girlfriend Sonia. At the same time, he could be very stubborn (which is absolutely a Scott family trait) and, at times, could flare up with anger if he got mad at something he did not agree with (yet another Scott family trait). He wasn't always direct with his love and would show it in different ways. Whenever you visited, he would go out and detail your car, making it look brand new. You didn't ask him to do it, but he would do it even if you tried to stop him. This was his passion.

My grandparents were having guests over one time and when they left, they walked right past their own car after it was detailed by Kevin. My grandfather saw his guests standing outside of his house looking around and asked what they were doing. The one guest finally recognized his car and was wondering how it got so clean. Kevin stepped up and said he just washed it. The man replied that he did more than just wash the car as it looked cleaner than it would have been sitting for sale at the dealership. Kevin was always proud to receive those types of reactions and compliments for his hard work and talent.

Late in the summer of '96 after his passing, I remember being cuddled in my dad's arms sitting by an apple tree we had in the backyard. I had tears running down my face because I was thinking about my nonno and uncle Kevin and their passing.

I asked my dad why we had to die; I didn't understand why it happened. My dad told me that everyone gets their turn one day. There's no discrimination of any sort; it was just in God's hands. He explained that Nonno's body had cancer that was like a weed that grew and overtook his body. My uncle Kevin was younger, but the answer was the same. Life continues even when someone gets very sick. As much as you love someone, you want the best for them and you don't want them to suffer in the end. It would be selfish to not let them go and be at peace.

I had to ask what I considered a big question for my age: "Am I going to die?" My dad gave it to me straight but promised that I had lots of time left. He also said that we keep our loved ones and their memories in our hearts and that they would want us to carry on living our lives to the fullest. This was the moment when I felt close to God and Jesus. I also felt like nonno and my uncle Kevin were present in spirit. From that day forward, I would feel it when anyone I loved was around me in spirit.

As time went on, I would pray in bed before going to sleep. I often had dreams about Jesus coming to me and healing my CP — *wouldn't that be nice*. When you're a child, you slowly become aware of your own mortality and situation, and you try to make sense of it as an adult would, so being in a Catholic school and learning about the Bible put religion and the idea of praying in my head. If I kept praying hard enough, I would be healed over time as I grew up. Of course, that's not how that works and you come to realize that over time, but it didn't stop me from dreaming about it. Who wouldn't wish for that?

Classic Nonna

On Saturday, October 29th, 2011, my nonna Maria D'Agostino peacefully passed away at the age of eighty-six of congestive heart failure. It was a day filled with mixed emotions. On one hand, we were celebrating the marriage of our cousin on my nonna's side. But on the other hand, my family had lost a mother, sister, aunt, cousin, friend and, most importantly, a nonna.

Back in 1999, three years after her husband passed away, she finally decided to move in with us because she didn't want to be alone. Everybody in the family except us knew this was happening. My parents found out through my uncle Joe and other cousins. My parents had invited her to live with us many times in the past, not wanting her to be alone, but she didn't want to budge. She would often call our house to ask my mom to run errands for her, like getting groceries, and to have her daughter over for the company, so we knew she was lonely. At any rate, we were relieved that she finally gave in.

We had a decent-sized carport that we converted into an apartment for Nonna. A neighbour and some of his friends helped build the extension. I liked watching them build it after I came home from school and would help hang their tools and stuff to be involved. No wonder I love designing houses. The apartment had a small living room, bathroom and bedroom, which attached onto our upstairs living room.

When Nonna finally moved in, there was a bit of an adjustment period for all of us, but we figured it out. She spent a lot of time with Stirling and me. It sounds stereotypical, but she would have a bowl of pasta with her homemade tomato sauce ready for us when we came home from school every day. She attended every sporting event we had and could always be seen cheering us on. Stirling and I spent a lot of our time in Nonna's living room. We would watch TV, often Italian programming, while she would knit. If she wasn't watching TV or cooking, she was baking up a storm. None of us ever went hungry.

Because my brother was a high-spirited kid and quite a handful, Nonna gave him the nickname "Stirlach and pitch." This might not make sense, but she stretched his name out so she would have something to relate to. It could have been rooted in Italian, I'm not sure, but she would use the word "pitch" to describe him getting into mischief. We just went with it and didn't question it.

When she was in her late seventies, she began to develop paranoia dementia, which meant that she believed everyone was against her, especially my mom. She was forgetting to turn the stove elements and water off, even going as far as accidentally flooding our bathroom, along with many other incidents. She would also get combative by accusing us of doing things we didn't actually do. My mom and nonna had a disagreement one day about something that wasn't true at all. We found out that she wasn't taking her pills anymore, which was why she was behaving this way. At this point, Nonna recognized the dangers of what was happening and decided to put herself into a retirement home after living with us for almost ten years. Once again, we didn't know until we received a phone call from the home saying there was room for her. Classic Nonna, she moved in and moved out without telling us. We all knew this was the best course of action. It took a year for my nonna to get used to the home, often saying how much she hated it and would rather live in our partially finished basement if she had to than continue staying there.

Nonna worked for McMaster University as a custodian for just under twenty years and was a very compassionate, kind and loving person who showed her love through cooking, baking and knitting. She loved spending time with her family and friends, especially her grandchildren. We all miss her every day and keep her in our hearts.

You're Released from Your Worldly Restrictions and Set Free to Fly in Heaven

On Tuesday, January 22nd, 2013, my dad's mom, Evelyn Scott, passed away at seventy-five years old, only seven days away from her seventy-sixth birthday, after battling a muscle disease called dermatomyositis for three years. We had a beautiful luncheon with all of our family and friends at the funeral home. Evelyn was known for being a bit of a klutz and was accident-prone. The twilight of her years saw many injuries and accidents, which were painful, but also sadistically funny to whoever saw it happen (the Scott family just has that sadistic sense of humour).

We invited our intermediate family back to the house after the interment to spend time together. My cousin Matthew's girlfriend (now wife) Ashley was with us. We brought out a folding table that she sat at with her drink. As she was talking, she leaned in and put some weight on the table, which then proceeded to collapse, sending her drink straight to the floor. I guess the table wasn't fully secured and locked in because that shouldn't have happened otherwise. I couldn't stop laughing because I was sitting right across from her and saw her face, almost in slow motion as it happened. I proudly dubbed Ashley the new Evelyn of the family. We spent the rest of the evening reminiscing about Evelyn and recounting her many accidents.

My grandma was an exceptional woman who would give up her life in a minute to save someone she loved. She had a very loving and uplifting personality; she loved to dance, laugh and have a good time. She absolutely adored her husband, Walter, and was very protective of him to the point of getting jealous whenever a woman asked him to dance or "try to steal him." All of us had to keep an eye on her if she was having a drink because her personality changed rather quickly as she became fairly belligerent.

Grandma always had a nickname for everyone. She often called people "cluckheads," and if she didn't know a lady's name, she would call them Alice or Doris. Why she picked those particular names is something we will never know.

As I mentioned earlier, my grandma was known for calamitous, self-induced injuries fit for a comedy routine. She fell off her bike into a ditch one time with my cousin Brittany. Tripped over a gopher hole and rolled down a hillside. Was stung to death when she tried sucking up bees and hornets with a vacuum. Slipped on the ice at a cemetery, which slid her under a parked car and broke her elbow. Tragically, she was also hit by a car at sixty-two years old, which required months of rehabilitation to recover as best as she could.

Grandma loved her costume jewellery — anything big, shiny, and sparkling. My uncle Gordon and Dad bought lots of bling as they say, over the years. She particularly loved a custom diamond ring my dad got her. She wore it every time she went out, especially on planes because she believed it got her better service. She pretended to be Mrs. Chancellor, the wealthy lady from the soap opera, the young and the restless, she was always "blinged" out.

Grandma worked as a custodian at the Hamilton-Wentworth District School Board for twenty-four years. We know she had a great life and there was never a dull moment with her around. She is greatly missed and may she rest in peace.

Kyle N. Scott

Carry On and Live Life:
A Tribute to Grandpa Scott

At the beginning of March 2014, we took my grandpa Scott (Walter) to Fallsview Casino in Niagara Falls for his seventy-eight birthday. Months earlier, we had also promised to take my aunt Anna for her birthday, which was back in October, so we made it up to her by bringing her along too. When my dad went in to get my grandpa, he said he was going to bring his cane, which he never uses. My dad found it odd but figured long-standing issues with my grandpa's back must have been progressing.

During our ride down to the casino, Anna must have said, "Your what hurts?" about a million times to my grandpa. She sometimes gets on these phrases and keeps saying them to annoy(ing) people. Both my grandpa and Anna knew each other well, but it didn't stop her from getting on his nerves. "I'll give her what hurts!" he said more than once, but my dad pressed him not to engage. "Don't wake the lion," as my dad would say.

At the casino, we noticed that Grandpa was out of breath after walking less than ten feet. With concern, my dad asked him what was going on with him. Grandpa was explaining that this was what he has been experiencing for the past several weeks, a shortness of breath. My dad immediately thought it could be lung cancer since my grandpa had smoked for most of his life. We stayed at the casino at his behest since he didn't want to ruin the outing. On the way home, my dad tried to convince him to go to the hospital to get some tests done. He declined and asked to be taken straight home, knowing full well that he should be in the hospital.

The next day, my grandpa came to his senses and decided to see his family doctor. My dad went with him to see what was going on. The doctor wasn't much help, citing that the previous lung x-ray seemed normal. My dad pointed out my grandpa's yellow neck; however, the doctor just gave him iron pills and some other ones to help him sleep. After they left, my dad begged him to get a full scan done at the hospital, not trusting that the doctor had done his job. Three days later, my grandpa was in the hospital receiving a battery of tests.

After being in the hospital for five days, test results were coming in and the doctor set up a meeting with the immediate family to give the bad news. My grandpa had stage four lung cancer, three large tumours, and adrenal and spinal cancer. He was a heavy smoker so it's highly possible that was one of the causes, if not the actual cause. The hospital doctor gave my grandpa roughly three months to live. "I won't last three months. It's more like three weeks," my grandpa said as the doctor left. After a long pause, he turned to my uncle Gordon and Dad to say, "Take out a paper and pencil, and start writing."

A few nights later, my dad and I went to visit him. A nurse came in to assist him and introduced herself. "Bee?" he responded, not sure if that's what he heard.

The nurse came right up to his face and loudly said, "It's Bead!"

Stunned, my grandpa shot back in his chair and said, "Lady, I may be old, but I'm not deaf!" My grandpa was known to tell it like it was. He was always funny about it, but people would take him the wrong way when he was actually just trying to be funny.

The nurse asked my grandpa how he got the name Walter. My dad popped in to speak for him, telling her that when his mother was asked for her son's name, she asked for water. The nurse thought she said Walter, which she wrote down as his name. Bead just said, "What a wonderful story," totally believing it to be true. My grandpa just shook his head.

The family repeatedly made the suggestion for Grandpa to transfer to a hospice, but he declined every time and demanded to spend his last days at home. When he was discharged from the hospital, the family took turns visiting the house each day to make sure he was okay and to share some laughs with him before he passed.

One evening, my dad, cousin Sharon who was a retired nurse (came up from North Carolina once she heard the news) and I were in the kitchen with Grandpa having a conversation. Out of nowhere, Grandpa started talking to the stove. "Hi Joe, long time no see. How are you doing?" We all looked at each other and thought the medicine must have really been kicking in. We asked him if he was alright and who Joe was. He turns with a blank expression on his face and says, "Who?" We told him that he was just talking to some guy named Joe. He couldn't keep a straight face as he tried to play it off like he was talking to the dead and started to laugh. "Gotcha!" No matter how much pain or discomfort he was feeling, my grandpa kept his wicked sense of humour until the very end.

A week before he passed, he was granted a 24-hour, in-home nurse. When we first met her, she knew exactly who my dad was because my grandpa must have been talking about him. She introduced herself as Feng, but she pronounced it as "Fung."

"I married a Scotsman too!" she said enthusiastically. My dad was curious and asked her what her last name was thinking it would be something like McCain, McDonald, or McCarthy. "It's Loo." Now, the word "vaffanculo" in Italian means "f**k you," and her name sounded awfully similar.

"If anyone ever asked for your name in Italy, like if you go to a hotel or something, and you say your name, they would immediately kick you out of the hotel," my dad told her. My grandpa just shook his head in disbelief, not understanding where this was going. My dad explained her name's similarity to the Italian swear word, which got her to laugh. My dad honestly thought he was saving her life by making her aware of the possible miscommunication stemming from her name.

Earlier in the week, we agreed to have my grandpa placed in hospice by April 7th. When the decision was made, he asked who would pay for his transportation costs. We said to use his credit card. "Well, I was going to save that money," he responded. My uncle Gordon laughed and said, "What, so we can all get $30 more in inheritance?"

The day before he passed, he asked my uncle Wayne, who was living with him at the time, if my dad would cut his hair that evening. Wayne said he would ask, and Grandpa replied, "Okay, good. I want to look good when I see Evelyn." We ordered pizza that night and enjoyed each other's company. Grandpa was in good spirits and doing what he usually does, making everyone laugh. After my dad finished his final haircut, my grandfather thanked him and washed dishes for the last time. Then he started to brush his teeth. He paused, looked back at us.

"Is everything alright?" we asked him.

"Do you guys mind? Jesus!" he shot back a little embarrassed. That was a classic Walter Scott response — sarcastic and witty.

On the morning of Sunday, April 6th, 2014, my grandpa Scott passed away peacefully at his family home of thirty-six years. The entire family had only seen him several hours before. His final thoughts were, "Carry on and live life."

With Us in Spirit: Tributes to Family and Friends Who Have Passed

Every time I was with my grandfather, he always made sure that he put a smile on my face. He loved making me laugh with his sarcastic stories and jokes. Besides being a jokester, he was also a self-taught musician, but could often be straightforward and didn't take any crap from anyone. I'll illustrate that with a quick story. He could play the piano as well as any professional pianist, but he did start out with lessons when he was younger. Piano teachers back in the day used to slam the piano key cover over your fingers when they felt like you weren't listening or taking the lesson seriously. My grandfather told his mom about it and she responded that he must have deserved it. He knew he had to take matters into his own hands. During his next lesson, he asked his teacher to show him how to play something, and while his teacher was playing, he slammed the cover down on her fingers, telling her to take their piano and shove it. He never went back but did apologize for doing it. He continued teaching himself from that day forward and went on to play at churches and other functions including our get-togethers.

He played pretty much right up until his passing. When he walked away from the piano after he played for the last time, he was emotional and claimed that it was his last time he would be able to play. That moment was very emotional for him and for all of us in attendance.

As a teenager, he was a cook at Martin's Steak House until he found a position at Silverwood's Dairy while starting and raising a family. Due to injuries he received while working as a dairy delivery driver, he took time off to heal before working for the Hamilton Street Railway (HSR) for the next twenty-three years.

He was a caregiver. He took care of my great-grandparents, his wife, and his son Kevin when he became sick. The family often thought he missed his calling as he would have made a wonderful nurse. We miss you and even though you were the glue that held the family together, we're all doing alright down here.

Marc, May the Force Be with You, Always

On Wednesday, July 12th, 2017, I lost one of my dearest friends, Marc, who lost his battle with cancer, but put up a valiant fight. He had a special zest for life and touched the hearts of everyone he met. He loved music, and singing and dancing to all the Disney movies. He had a passion for Star Wars, the Toronto Blue Jays and Maple Leafs, and the Hamilton Tiger-Cats. Not only did Marc and I attend St. Thomas More together, but we also played baseball and sledge hockey on the same team as well; he was an excellent goaltender. Each time he saved a goal, he would always yell out, "I saved the puck!" like he was surprised.

Marc had many medical challenges in his life, but he met them all with a constant smile and ever-present good manners. Rest in peace, Marc. We all miss you! May the Force be with you!

A Devastating Loss of Aunt Susu

Late on Thursday, February 21st, 2019, my aunt Susan passed away. My family received a group message from her only son, my cousin Matthew, stating that he hadn't heard from her in a few days. He lived out of town and wasn't able to physically check on her. My aunt Ruth and her friend went to the house after receiving the message only to confirm our worst fears. Sadly, she had to be alone in her final moments because she had been living alone for the past year, ever since her husband, Michael, passed away from ALS. Their departures were only a year and three days apart from each other.

Susan had a fun and loving personality, with a love for children and especially her son, Matthew. She struggled with serious mental health issues, which led to her diabetes getting out of control, ultimately leading to her death. She was mischievous at times and would often cause drama with family members over the years. I can honestly say that there was never a dull moment with her around because she was always up to something or saying such bizarre things.

Even though I mostly saw my aunt at family gatherings, I always had a great relationship with her. We shared many waves of laughter and stories throughout the years. I was always entertained by her, what was she going to come up with next.

We had a double service for Mike and Susan — a two-for-one special as my cousin jokingly called it. Matthew held onto his father's ashes from the previous year for personal reasons, but also feeling that something like this would happen to his mother after she lost her husband. Matthew and our family, especially my dad, tried their best to help Susan before it was too late, but she was never receptive. Even the health care system failed her in the end, which makes the whole situation even sadder. She didn't stand much of a chance and it opened a lot of our eyes to the realities of mental illness.

I thought Matthew's full eulogy that he gave at the funeral summarized his parents' relationship quite well, and I wanted to share a piece of it in this book to help paint a better picture of who my aunt Susan was.

> Thank you everyone for coming today. It really means a lot to my family and especially to me.
>
> Trying to distill the thirty-five years I knew my parents into an engaging five-minute speech was a difficult task. I could have written a three-part epic that would encompass all the laughter, sadness, and insanity that surrounded their existence. Fortunately, I can spare you the trouble because I am happy to announce that I just signed a deal with Netflix to produce a multi-season TV show called "I Love You, I'll Kill You," a fictional story inspired by my parents' marriage. That was my parents: two people married by law, but lovingly at each other's throats by choice with me as the referee.
>
> Those of us who knew Susan would agree that she was the mischievous perpetrator of nearly every source of drama she was involved in. Sometimes she got caught, other times she got away with it. She often found humour in inappropriate things and marched to the beat of her own drum, and she would beat it to antagonize the cats she loved so very much. The quickest way to summarize who my mother was is to tell you a story that took place when I was eleven years old.
>
> While at a neighbour's house, my mother took it upon herself to brazenly take an egg from their own fridge, walk out into their backyard and throw it at their back window. She then proceeded

to walk around the house and re-enter from the front as if nothing happened. The neighbours ran into the backyard looking for the vandal, never catching a glimpse because that vandal was standing right behind them in the house asking, "What the heck happened?"

I can only hope my "Aunt Susu" is happy in Heaven and has been reunited with her late husband, Mike.

Claudio, the Theatre Man!

On Monday, June 29th, 2020, my family and I received one of the most devastating phone calls we could ever have received. The call was about my cousin Claudio who passed away from a heart attack at work. What a shock! No one had a clue — including, most likely, Claude himself — that he had any health issues at all. He was only fifty-six years old. He was my second cousin on my mother's side and was one of the most charismatic people I have ever known. Needless to say, my family will go through a long adjustment period as we get used to Claudio's absence at family events.

I cannot express the sorrow I felt when we got that phone call and I'll be mourning the loss for quite some time. It will never be the same when we have our family events without having him provide so many laughs. However, I know he will always be there with all of us in spirit because he was always devoted to his family, relatives and friends. He enjoyed the simple things in life. Claudio loved pizza, pasta, wine and espresso. Actually, he simply loved life as a whole. He would always listen to you and was always willing to try new things. He never wanted to bother anyone, so much so that at times he would disappear, and no one could get a hold of him. Sometimes we thought of putting a GPS tracker on him just to make sure he was around. He was always present whenever you needed him, though. He never missed a family event and if you were sick, he would come to visit to check if you needed anything or just to talk and laugh. He was always present even in the hardest of times.

People would ask how he could always smile and how he managed to always be happy. His answer, of course, was always the same joke. "'Cause I'm not married!" and he would laugh out loud as only he could. He was a man who embraced life in a way that I have never seen and dedicated his life to his family and friends. I never saw him get angry, I never even heard him raise his voice outside of his normal, boisterous nature. He never spoke ill of anyone and didn't have a jealous bone in his body. He was the most genuine person I have ever met, and he was never focused on what people thought of him. Instead, he was focused on making sure everyone around him was okay.

Claudio was a great guy with a huge laugh and a heart of gold! He particularly loved his family and friends, and had a passion for theatre. He loved nothing better than to get dressed up, go out for a nice dinner (or lunch, for those matinees), and then catch a live performance.

He loved going to see plays, musicals, and Broadway shows at the theatre. It didn't matter if he saw it ten times over; he always acted like it was his first time. He attended every show you could ever imagine, all over Ontario: Hamilton, Niagara-on-the-Lake, Toronto, St. Jacobs, Stratford, and all the small cities in between on weekdays, but mostly on weekends when there wasn't a family event. This is why I called him "Claudio the Theatre Man."

To honour my cousin Claudio's memory, my entire family wants to do something that would have meant a lot to him instead of having flowers at his funeral. It's something he wanted to do himself but didn't get the chance. We want to have a plaque made saying "In Memory of Claudio D'Alessio" and have it affixed on theatre chairs across the Greater Toronto Area. We all know that Claudio was always devoted to every family event that was held and continues to be in spirit; however, we also know where he is when there are no family events — at the theatre in his pledged seat. If you happen to see a play in the future, keep an eye out for his chair. The chair might not be cheap, but you're more than welcome to take a picture in it for free!

In October 2020, just before Canadian Thanksgiving, the D'Alessio family received an email from Claudio's colleagues at Aerloc Industries with a picture of a bench he used to sit at during his lunch breaks. The bench now had a plaque saying, "In Memory of Claudio D'Alessio – Colleague & Friend" with an image of wire pliers he used to work with. His bench is located at the corner of Mercer and Head Street in Dundas, Ontario. If you live in the area or find yourself there one day, feel free to visit for a little peace and quiet. Just make sure you don't go during work hours in case they are wondering why a stranger is randomly sitting in Claudio's spot.

Claudio was never technologically savvy. He didn't want anything to do with computers or cell phones. A little over a decade ago, his family bought him a computer, hoping it would encourage him to keep up with the times. It seemed to work for a while until he started having issues with both the machine and the Internet. I can't recall exactly, but he always had some excuse for not using it. Hey, that was Claudio. How can you not have a cell phone in this day and age? Well, he said, and I quote, "There's no chance in hell that I'm getting a cell phone." There's certainly no other way to interpret that statement.

About seven or eight years ago, Claudio was over on the morning of Christmas Eve for a visit before heading to one of his sisters for their Christmas tradition — and they are a big family, more thirty in just their family alone. He said, "Kyle, I got this gut feeling that my family got me a stupid cell phone."

I laughed and asked, "Why do you think that?" knowing that they already told me about it.

"Because they keep hounding me to get one, thinking that they can get a hold of me faster... pfft... I will turn it off. I don't want anyone to know where I am or bug me," Claudio added.

I said, "Well, maybe they want to make sure that you don't drop off the face of the Earth."

His answer was, "Don't worry, I'm okay... everyone worries too much." Literally a minute later, as Claudio was reaching for something out of his pocket, he said, "Kyle, guess what?! I got a cellphone." A flip one for $18 per month...

Now, I'm laughing my head off, trying not to fall off my wheelchair and knowing he has not one, but two cell phones. He was laughing hysterically, saying, "Wait until I show them this!" Once again, that was my cousin Claudio.

He was a traditional, old-fashioned guy. If you wanted to talk to him, you had to call him on a landline and you wouldn't be guaranteed to get him even if he was at home. If you left a message, you had to leave an important one, otherwise, he wouldn't call back. If you saw him at a family occasion and enquired about your message, he would just say, "Yes," meaning he got it. Of course, the next thing you ask is why he didn't call you back, and he would say, "Well, it wasn't that important." Again, that was Claudio. If you did manage to get him on the phone, we would write it down on the calendar like it was a momentous occasion. If you ever asked him what he was doing, one of his famous responses was, "Talking to you! What are you doing?"

Claudio was known for his sayings. Here are a few of my favourites.

- When Claudio was working with his father, they would sometimes get into disagreements. Claudio's father, in anger, would say that he wouldn't last thirty minutes working for him in construction. Claudio would quickly reply that he "would quit after fifteen minutes."
- "I stand here, you stand there." He jokingly said this to a woman he was dating after she asked him where they stood in the relationship.
- "It's not too shabby." Meaning, things worked out well.
- "It needs a little bit of elbow grease." Since he was a landlord with his cousin, he would say this after cleaning a stove full of grease that a tenant had never cleaned.
- "Aiutami Dice" in Italian means "help me say it." He would say this if someone said something that supported his position or argument.
- "Who are those guys?" It's a quote taken from *Butch Cassidy and the Sundance Kid*, an old Robert Redford and Paul Newman movie. Claudio liked to use it when they were moving along quickly finishing a job.
- "Kyle, will you be my best man at my wedding?" Yes, I said and asked him who was the special lady, knowing he had some sort of joke behind it. "Well, I gotta find her first and ask her, then I will let you know!"
- "*Hai capito*," which means, "Did you understand?" (Italian dialect). However, Claudio would use the Fondi's dialect leaving out the ending of the words. In Claudio's dialect, he would say "hai capeet," using the typical Italian hand gestures to go along with it, of course.

Claudio was an honest and hard worker and worked at Dominion Glass, Robinson Steel and Aerloc Industries as a crane operator for years. However, he would come up with any excuse not to go into work. He would tell his boss that he was sick when he didn't want to go into work, so he could play hooky. There was a time when he didn't go into work for two weeks because he didn't feel like it. He didn't even call in sick; he just didn't show up. After a few weeks, his work called the family out of concern to see where he was. Work even called his house, but as I've mentioned, he didn't pick up the phone, again saying he didn't want to talk to them. Who does that? One of his excuses that I can remember was that he "hit a snowbank," which damaged his car. The other one was claiming that a skunk had sprayed him, which was suggested by my dad and me.

Death is a reality we all must face, and it was something Claudio understood very clearly. When we talked about death, he would always say to me, "You know, when it's your time to go, you gotta go! Dat's all!" He did not like to focus on the negatives; he lived very much for the present and tried to enjoy the moment. At every funeral and as a constant visitor of the cemetery, he would always say, "You know... people are dying to get into this place," and again he would laugh. He was always smiling, and his laugh was so unique and infectious it would draw attention even in the loudest room.

Claudio was taken away from us far too soon. He will be truly missed by his family, numerous aunts and uncles, relatives and friends, and will always be remembered for being a character. He once said, "You can't be afraid to die. We all have to exit sometime."

Peace is in You, Mr. Pizza

On the evening of Saturday, January 9th, 2021, my family and I lost one of our special family friends Glen, at the age of seventy, after battling cancer that returned three and a half years later.

As you have read, Glen, also known as Mr. Pizza is the husband of the titanium queen, Laura — Ya-Ya. They have been friends of our family for many years. In my thirty-one years, I have been blessed to have Mr. Pizza a part of my life. We have so many wonderful memories and laughs that

With Us in Spirit: Tributes to Family and Friends Who Have Passed

will stay with us for a lifetime. I will always embrace the strength of the man that he was. He has taught me in silent ways how to be kind and to be a gentleman. Mr. Pizza once said to me that, "you are only responsible for yourself, nobody else." This will be the phrase of wisdom that I will carry throughout my life in memory of him.

In 1971, Glen join the Hamilton Fire Department where he rose through the ranks and after twenty-five years, left Hamilton to become the Fire Chief of Burlington, where he remained until 1999. Glen was recruited to return to Hamilton as Chief to lead the Fire and EMS Services through the amalgamation process of seven local governments to the new City of Hamilton. This amalgamation created not only one of the largest composite Fire Services in Canada, but one of Canada's highest rated. Glen's tenure in Emergency Services was followed by positions in senior management culminating in him becoming Hamilton's City Manager (CAO) for the last five years of his municipal service. On leaving the city, Glen taught at the college level, lectured across Canada and provided consultant services. October 2009, Glen was appointed to the Ontario Court of Justice where he remained a Justice of the Peace until his death. Glen praised the knowledge, commitment and dedication of those in the Justice System as they served the citizens of Ontario.

Glen was a hard-working, respected, esteemed, family man who served his community for fifty years as a Firefighter, Fire Chief, City Manager of Hamilton and Justice of the Peace.

Glen was an extraordinary gentleman who was compassionate, caring and well respected by everyone. I consider myself fortunate to have Mr. Pizza as my friend.

One less peace in the world… it's what we need more of.

"PEACE," be with you!

In everybody's lifetime, we lose the people we love who were a part of our journey and holds a special place in our hearts. However, goodbyes are not forever, they are not the end; it simply means I'll miss you until we meet again!

Chapter 14: Poetic Musings

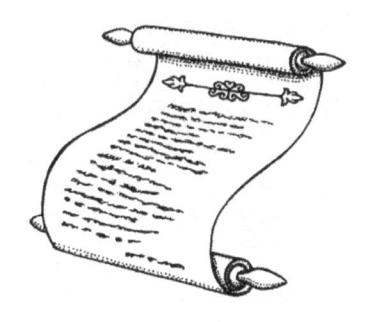

As I wrap up the book, I just wanted to share these poems I've written with you.

Make My World Shine

Love is a joy that fills my heart,
It strengthens me inside.
Love is a feeling I want to share,
My search roams far and wide.
I'm hunting for that one true love,
Whose hands will be holding mine.
I look for someone who will be holding me,
Sharing, caring, feeling safe inside.
The woman I love will share my thoughts,
Our dreams will intertwine.
Love is everything to me,
With love, the whole world will truly shine.

Kyle N. Scott

What Do You See?

What do you see when you look at me?
Do you see my beautiful eyes?
Are you attracted to my witty charm?
Or do you see me and only cry?
What do you see when you look at me?
Do you see beyond the chair?
Do you hear the words I'm saying to you?
Or do you see more than you can bear?
What do you see when you look at me?
Will you take the time to see the inner man?
Would you dare to see beyond the chair,
And find the sensitive man?
What do you see when you look at me?
I watch as you stare with curious fears,
And hear your mocking taunts.
Do you think I can't hear your hurtful jeers?
What do you see when you look at me?
Here I am! I am me!
I love, I laugh, I celebrate.
I tell jokes to make you laugh with glee!
What do you see when you look at me?
My rise to greatness lies within.
My inspiration comes from up high.
Look inside the disabled man, beyond the skin.

Poetic Musings

What Would Make Me the Happiest Guy on Earth?

I want to be able to wake up in the morning to the woman I love.
Be able to check on her, say, "Good morning, sweetheart," and give a soft and sweet kiss.
A woman who is willing to lay in bed on a Sunday, talk and laugh for hours.
Make pancakes, waffles and bacon together, be silly and have a good time.
A woman who can see beyond this disabled body of mine, who makes me feel good emotionally and physically.
Someone I can be cheesy and romantic with, showing my affections and feelings.
A woman who plays music and dances with me in my wheelchair while in the kitchen.
Someone who supports me, no matter what and is my biggest cheerleader.
A woman who's willing to try new adventures and share her dreams.
Someone who will always be by my side with family and friends as I stand by hers.
A woman who will be the mother of my children.
Someone who will grow old with me.
A woman who would make me the happiest guy on Earth,
Because that woman would show me what true love is.

Kyle N. Scott

What If I Didn't Have Cerebral Palsy?

What if I wasn't born with CP?
Where would I be?
It wouldn't have changed my personality,
But it would change me physically.
Could I run faster than I can move in my power wheelchair?
Would I race for the gold medal?
Would I be driving my lime-green car that would catch everyone's eye as I drive by?
Rather than getting a speeding ticket in my wheelchair.
I would go on adventures, hikes, to beaches, and climb stairs,
Instead of always finding another way around.
Would I speak any clearer than I already do?
Or would people still have trouble following me?
When I play sports, would I have full control and precision?
Would I move around unaided and be a dependable part of the team?
Would I have had more girls dance with me because they wanted to,
And not because they pity a man in a wheelchair?
Would all of the pretty girls go out with me?
Or would I still be left behind and unwanted?
Where would I have studied? Would I have left the city?
Would I still be an architectural technician or in another profession?
Would I own a house alone or with someone else?
Would I have married and started a family before thirty?
What could have been if I weren't disabled?
What could I have been without cerebral palsy?

My World Is My Wheels

There's been a wheelchair following me,
Since I lost my ability to walk.
It follows me on all occasions,
It doesn't matter what time is on the clock.
It's there in the morning for breakfast,
And it's there in the evening when I dine.
This wheelchair following me is not underfoot,
Worse, it is under my behind.
When I meet friends for lunch,
I always worry about finding a seat.
Ah, but wait just a minute,
This wheelchair has already swept me off my feet.
Sometimes my mind plays tricks on me,
It feels like someone else is pushing my chair.
I often want to stand up and run,
Scream "I'm healed!" just to give everyone a scare.
My world is my wheels,
Of that, I have no doubt.
They take me where I need to go,
And they help me get about.

Kyle N. Scott

What Do You Really Want in a Man?

I have to find someone who is open to my disability. All it will take is that one special woman who will see me for me.

If I say no woman wants to date a person with a disability, am I being too harsh or realistic about it?

They say, "This isn't really about you having CP," or "That's not true all." And tell me, "You're a kind, sweet, caring and funny man."

"You're the perfect image of what a man should be." So, really, what's the scoop?

Well, let's be realistic here. I get it, no one wants to date a disabled person. Or even want to be disabled themselves because it changes things.

However, what does everyone really want? Someone to love and make them feel good. To be happy, to laugh and appreciate life?

Or someone who takes advantage of that love and causes drama? What do people really want?

A physical or personal connection? Are you attracted to a body you can touch or a personality you can connect with?

Maybe it's both or one or the other, who am I to say? I know for darn sure though that finding a decent guy isn't always in the cards, so why not take a chance on me?

Music plays a big part in my life. I listen to music when I need inspiration, when I need support and when I want to relax. Since I can't have all of my favourite songs in my book, I wanted to include one song that's very heartfelt and inspirational to me. The message that I got from this song was telling me to try cause if I don't... I will never win. Hopefully, you will feel the impact as I did. This is a song written and sang by the country music icon Dolly Parton in 2014. Courtesy of The Dollywood Foundation.

Try

I have chased after rainbows
I've captured one or two
I've reached for the stars
I've even held a few
I've walked that lonesome valley
Topped the mountains, soared the sky
I've laughed and I have cried
But I have always tried

I've always been a dreamer
And dreams are special things
But dreams are of no value
If they're not equipped with wings
So secure yourself for climbing
Make ready for the flight
Don't let your chance go by
You'll make it if you try

So try to be the first one up the mountain
And try to be the first to touch the sky
And try to be one that make a difference
Try to put your fear and doubt aside

And try to make the most of every moment
'Cause if you never try you never win
So try each day to try a little harder
And if you fall, get up and try again

Nothing is impossible
If you can just believe
Don't live your life in shackles
When faith can be the key
The winner's one that keeps determination in his eyes
Who's not afraid to fly and not afraid to try

Kyle N. Scott

So try to be the first one up that mountain
And try to be the first to touch the sky
And try to count your blessings and keep counting
And try to soar where only eagles fly

And if you fail at first just keep on trying
For you are not a failure in God's eyes
The first step is the one that's always hardest
But you won't amount too much if you won't try
So spread your wings and let the magic happen
'Cause you'll never really know if you don't try

You gotta try
Come give it a try
You have to try
I know it ain't easy, who ever said it was
Life is hard, same as it ever was
You have to try

When you think you can't do it just try a little harder
Just dig a little deeper and go a little further but try
You have to try

What every it is you're gonna get through it
Let the spirit lead you I know you can do it
Just try
Just give it a try
And whenever you think you ain't gonna make
Put a smile on your face, suck it up and take it for a while
At least you know you tried

Don't think that I don't suffer
I know what I'm saying
When I get to that place where I start praying
And I try
Lord knows I try
Yes I try

Epilogue

Personally, I would like to thank everyone who has supported me and taken the time to read this book. For nearly a decade, I have hinted to my closest friends and family that I had always wanted to write a book, but I never imagined that it would become a reality. In 2016, I started writing the book but gave up too soon. I suppose I wasn't ready back then and needed time to figure out what the book would be. In January 2019, I vowed to myself that I would not stop typing until the book was completed! And here it is, the book in your hands right now. I was so inspired by writing it that I have created a children's illustration book and hopefully that will be published in the future! With that said, I really hope you enjoy the book because I poured my blood, sweat and tears into it; I put many hours thinking and planning what I wanted to say and how I wanted to express my thoughts.

My goal from the beginning was to express my feelings in words and to give you insight into my life in a positive but realistic manner. I hope you agree that I've achieved that. I wanted to write this book not only to share my experiences living with a disability but also to educate others on what daily life is like with cerebral palsy and to let those struggling with their own challenges know that they are not alone in their frustrations. It's OKAY to be unique or different, but don't let that interfere with your dreams and goals.

Despite the frustrations and obstacles that I have faced over the years, I am still immensely proud of all that I have accomplished over the past thirty years. I am proud of the opportunities I have created for myself and the occasions when I made all the troubles into opportunities.

I hope this book inspires someone with a disability, especially the younger generation. We've come a long way generationally in terms of understanding what it means to be disabled, but I believe we still have a long way to go. Anyone's life can change in a split second, but it's all about how you take control and your ability to turn it into something spectacular.

Just like you, I always had a vision of what my life was supposed to be like, but I was given a unique role to play by God. Remember when I mentioned that God has plans for me? Well, maybe this is just the beginning of them!

As a result of writing this book, I learned what I would like to do in the future, but before I do that, there is one thing I absolutely want from life, which is to find love and be married with children of my own.

After spending so much time researching organizations that help disabled individuals experience their bodies, I discovered a major gap in coverage within Canada. Typically these organizations are located in the United States, but British Columbia appears to be the only hub in Canada where they are offered — *I want to change that.* One of my goals is to bring the same opportunities here in Ontario because I strongly believe that every adult, regardless of physical disability, challenge or injury, has the right to explore themselves and experience intimacy, self-love and full humanness. Successfully implementing something like this would be a dream come true and an absolute accomplishment. Imagine lives it would change. My second goal is to establish a charity fund that will assist people with cerebral palsy get the equipment and devices they need to succeed in the world! My third goal... maybe it's a dream, a dream that could be a possibility is to build a Health and Wellness Centre. I realize what it takes to build such a facility, however, it resonates in my daily thoughts and I am passionate about it. This facility would be for people with CP as well as other disabilities. There would be a swimming pool with a hydrotherapy spa, exercise room, massage therapy and physiotherapy. This would give us more opportunities to socialize and network amongst ourselves and our support workers. This outlet could enable some if they wish, they may find that special person in their life — *you never know, where it may lead.*

Another goal, dreaming of course, would be to get on a reality talk show. I would be beyond grateful to even be in the audience, which wouldn't be a bad option considering how much I dislike being the centre of attention. Being on camera would be tough because I would be nervous and my spasticity would act up, causing me to lose control. I would be mortified. However, if the opportunity arose, I would do what I had to and find ways to keep everything under control because I wouldn't want to miss out on such an amazing opportunity. Who knows... if this book is a success, I may have the chance to appear on one of the Canadian talk shows. Depending on the success of the book, it might be featured on the Live with Kelly & Ryan in New York City or maybe somewhere like Los Angeles, The Late, Late Show with James Corden, heck, why not Jimmy Kimmel Live! too so I can meet his always-entertaining Aunt Chippy. She's so direct and has a spunky personality as I do. Maybe, just maybe The Ellen DeGeneres Show since she'll be ending her talk show after nineteen years. How awesome would it be if I appeared on her show and discussed my book?

Am I dreaming too big? Maybe. However, you are never too late to follow your dreams. In my wildest dream, maybe this could end up being a Netflix limited series or movie. If I'm going to dream, why not dream big. What would I title it as? Well, that's a tale for another time.

If you're going to do something, do it right. I've always been told, and sometimes, criticized for, how average I can be. I choose to ignore those words and instead tell myself every single day to shoot for the stars, to be the best I can be. Good enough isn't good enough if it can be better and better isn't better if it can be the best.

As I close out my book, I want to tell one final story that will bring everything into focus. Wisdom will come to you from the unlikeliest of sources and more often than not, that source is a failure. When you hit rock bottom, remember this. While you're struggling, that rocky, stable bottom can be a great foundation to build on and nurture personal growth. I'm not worried about whether the people I love will be successful. I'm worried they won't fail from time to time to learn something. A person who gets up off the floor and keeps growing, that's the person who continues to grow their influence throughout life.

Pick yourself up, dig your feet in and just stand up. No matter how rough the sea gets, you keep standing. You let the waves crash against your body and you persevere no matter what — *you never give up!*

What matters most to me is how I live, not what I have or do not have.

Let me ask you all one question, one that I have asked myself all my life: "How are you living?" Every day, ask yourself that question and reflect on it.

Need some ideas? Don't judge people or situations so quickly. Show up early with a smile on your face. Be kind. See how you can help make things better. Lend a hand. Dedicate yourself to doing things the right way. Don't be afraid to do what's right. Make an impact on your own and everyone else's life.

Thinking in this way will honour all those who have invested in you and those you've crossed paths with. Look in the unlikeliest places for that wisdom. Enhance your life every day by asking yourself, "How am I living?"

My sincere blessings to you all!

Thank you.

Author's Note

When writing this book, I thought a lot about how I could include everyone who has been a part of my journey and believe me, there are more stories than I can count and more people to thank. If you're not in this book, trust me, you're always in my heart. I tried my best to include them all but I would be writing forever. This book would have been 777 pages…

Since this proved to be impossible, I asked family and friends to share a personal message with me about our journey together. The response was overwhelming and heartwarming, and their messages have been included on my website to share with the world in the "Memories" section.

Please visit my website at kylenscott.ca and feel free to write a personal message of your own on the Readers' Thoughts. I look forward to reading any thoughts, reflections, and impressions that you may have after reading the book.

CPSIA information can be obtained
at www.ICGtesting.com
Printed in the USA
BVHW031533121221
623847BV00004B/8/J